EXPERT LPN GUIDES

I.V. Therapy

EXPERT LPN GUIDES

I.V. Therapy

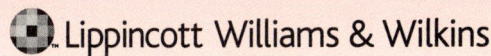 Lippincott Williams & Wilkins
a Wolters Kluwer business
Philadelphia · Baltimore · New York · London
Buenos Aires · Hong Kong · Sydney · Tokyo

STAFF

EXECUTIVE PUBLISHER
Judith A. Schilling McCann,
RN, MSN

EDITORIAL DIRECTOR
William J. Kelly

CLINICAL DIRECTOR
Joan M. Robinson, RN, MSN

SENIOR ART DIRECTOR
Arlene Putterman

EDITORIAL PROJECT MANAGER
Christiane L. Brownell, ELS

CLINICAL PROJECT MANAGER
Beverly Ann Tscheschlog, RN, BS

EDITORS
Toby Brener, Jon Zonderman

CLINICAL EDITOR
Anita Lockhart, RN, MSN

COPY EDITORS
Heather Ditch, Amy Furman,
Dona Perkins

DESIGNERS
Debra Moloshok (book design),
Jan Greenberg (project manager)

DIGITAL COMPOSITION SERVICES
Diane Paluba (manager),
Joyce Rossi Biletz; Donna S. Morris

MANUFACTURING
Patricia K. Dorshaw (director),
Beth J. Welsh

EDITORIAL ASSISTANTS
Megan L. Aldinger,
Karen J. Kirk, Linda K. Ruhf

DESIGN ASSISTANT
Georg Purvis 4th

INDEXER
Dianne Schneider

The clinical treatments described and recommended in this publication are based on research and consultation with nursing, medical, and legal authorities. To the best of our knowledge, these procedures reflect currently accepted practice. Nevertheless, they can't be considered absolute and universal recommendations. For individual applications, all recommendations must be considered in light of the patient's clinical condition and, before administration of new or infrequently used drugs, in light of the latest package-insert information. The authors and publisher disclaim any responsibility for any adverse effects resulting from the suggested procedures, from any undetected errors, or from the reader's misunderstanding of the text.

© 2007 by Lippincott Williams & Wilkins. All rights reserved. This book is protected by copyright. No part of it may be reproduced, stored in a retrieval system, or transmitted, in any form or by any means—electronic, mechanical, photocopy, recording, or otherwise—without prior written permission of the publisher, except for brief quotations embodied in critical articles and reviews and testing and evaluation materials provided by the publisher to instructors whose schools have adopted its accompanying textbook. Printed in the United States of America. For information, write Lippincott Williams & Wilkins, 323 Norristown Road, Suite 200, Ambler, PA 19002-2756.

LPNIV010306

Library of Congress Cataloging-in-Publication Data

LPN expert guides. I.V. therapy.
   p. ; cm.
  Includes bibliographical references and index.
  1. Intravenous therapy—Handbooks, manuals, etc. 2. Practical nursing—Handbooks, manuals, etc. I. Lippincott Williams & Wilkins. II. Title: I.V. therapy.
  [DNLM: 1. Infusions, Intravenous—methods—Handbooks. 2. Drug Therapy—methods—Handbooks. 3. Nursing, Practical—methods—Handbooks.
WY 49 L924 2007]
RM170.L66 2007
615'.6—dc22   2005034037
ISBN 1-58255-868-X (alk. paper)

Contents

	Contributors and consultants	vii
1	Introduction to I.V. therapy	1
2	Peripheral I.V. therapy	35
3	Central venous therapy	86
4	Administering I.V. drugs	149
5	Transfusions	194
6	Chemotherapy infusions	229
7	Parenteral nutrition	253
	Dangerous abbreviations	284
	Using a flow sheet to document I.V therapy	285
	Common fluid and electrolyte imbalances in children	286
	Common fluid and electrolyte imbalances in eldery patients	289
	Selected references	292
	Index	294

Contributors and consultants

Katrina D. Allen, RN, MSN, CCRN
Nursing Instructor
Faulkner State Community College
Bay Minette, Ala.

Penny Bennett, BSN
Owner
Instruction by Penny
Tyler (Tex.) Junior College

Janice W. Chapman, RN, MSN
Health Careers Site Coordinator & Instructor, School of Nursing
Reid State College
Atmore, Ala.

Tricia Duff, LPN, I.V. Certified
Coumadin Nurse
Concord (N.H.) Hospital

Diana Duffy, RN, BSN, MEd
PN Director, Health Careers Education Coordinator
Chisholm Trail Technology Center
Omega, Okla.

Renee D. Poling, LPN, AA, I.V. Certified
Charge Nurse
Traditions Care Center
Cleveland

Dina Nicole Salvatore, LPN
Charge Nurse
Windemere Nursing & Rehabilitation Center
Oak Bluffs, Mass.

1

INTRODUCTION TO I.V. THERAPY

Why I.V. therapy?

One of your most important nursing responsibilities is to give fluids to patients. In I.V. therapy, liquid solutions are introduced directly into the bloodstream.

I.V. therapy fulfills these main objectives:
- to restore and maintain fluid and electrolyte balance
- to administer drugs
- to transfuse blood and blood products
- to deliver parenteral nutrients and nutritional supplements.

(See *Benefits and risks of I.V. therapy*, page 2.)

TO RESTORE AND MAINTAIN FLUID AND ELECTROLYTE BALANCE

To understand how I.V. therapy works to restore fluid and electrolyte balance, let's first review some basics of fluids and electrolytes. The human body is composed largely of fluids. Fluids account for about two-thirds of total body weight in an average-sized adult who weighs 155 lb (70.3 kg) and for about three-fourths of total body weight in an infant.

Body fluids are composed of water (a solvent) and dissolved substances (solutes). The solutes in body fluids include electrolytes such as sodium and nonelectrolytes such as proteins.

Fluids

Body fluids fill these needs:
- help to regulate body temperature
- transport nutrients and gases throughout the body
- carry wastes to excretion sites
- maintain cell shape.

Benefits and risks of I.V. therapy

WHAT ARE THE BENEFITS?
- I.V. therapy can be used to give fluids, drugs, nutrients, and other solutions when a patient is unable to take these substances by mouth.
- I.V. drug delivery allows more accurate dosing.
- Because the entire amount of a drug reaches the bloodstream immediately, the drug begins to act almost instantaneously.

WHAT ARE THE RISKS?
- Like other invasive procedures, I.V. therapy carries risks, such as:
 – bleeding
 – infiltration (infusion of the I.V. solution into surrounding tissues rather than the blood vessel)
 – infection
 – overdose (because response to I.V. drugs is more rapid)
 – incompatibility when drugs and I.V. solutions are mixed
 – adverse or allergic reactions to an infused substance.
- When the patient must cope with I.V. poles, I.V. lines, and dressings, simple activity, such as transferring to a chair, walking, and washing, can become complicated.
- I.V. therapy is more costly than oral, subcutaneous, or I.M. therapies.

When fluid levels are correct, the body performs optimally, but when fluid levels fall above or below the acceptable range, organs and systems can quickly become impaired.

Body fluids exist in two major compartments: inside the cells and outside the cells. The fluid inside cells — about 55% of the total body fluid — is called *intracellular fluid* (ICF); the rest is called *extracellular fluid* (ECF). Normally, the distribution of fluids between the two compartments is constant. (See *Understanding body fluid distribution*.)

ECF occurs in two forms: interstitial fluid (ISF) and intravascular fluid. ISF surrounds each cell in the body; even bone cells are bathed in it. Intravascular fluid is blood plasma, the liquid component of blood. It surrounds red blood cells and accounts for most blood volume.

In an adult, about 5% of the body fluid is intravascular ECF, and about 15% is interstitial ECF. Part of that interstitial ECF is transcellular fluid, which includes cerebrospinal fluid and lymph. Transcellular fluid is found in the pleural and abdominal cavities.

The kidneys, heart, liver, adrenal and pituitary glands, and nervous system are all involved in maintaining fluid balance. Fluid balance is affected by:

Understanding body fluid distribution

Body fluid is distributed between two main compartments—extracellular and intracellular. Extracellular fluid (ECF) has two components—interstitial fluid (ISF) and intravascular fluid (plasma). This illustration shows body fluid distribution for a 155-lb (70.3-kg) adult.

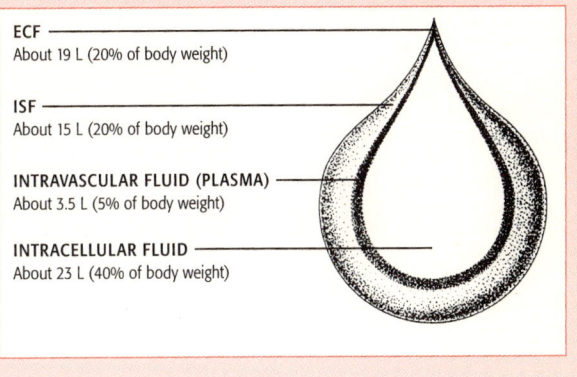

ECF
About 19 L (20% of body weight)

ISF
About 15 L (20% of body weight)

INTRAVASCULAR FLUID (PLASMA)
About 3.5 L (5% of body weight)

INTRACELLULAR FLUID
About 23 L (40% of body weight)

- concentration of solutes in the fluid
- distribution of fluids in the body
- fluid volume.

Every day, the body gains and loses fluid. To maintain fluid balance, the gains must equal the losses. (See *Daily fluid gains and losses,* page 4.)

Because a change of about 1 L of fluids changes weight about 2.2 lb (1 kg = 1 L = 2.2 lb), changes in fluid balance are best determined by daily weights.

Fluid volume and concentration are regulated by the interaction of two hormones: antidiuretic hormone (ADH) and aldosterone.

ADH affects fluid volume and concentration by regulating water retention and is secreted when plasma osmolarity (solute concentration) increases or circulating blood volume decreases and blood pressure drops. Aldosterone acts to retain sodium and water and is secreted when serum sodium is low, potassium is high, or the circulating volume of fluid decreases.

> ## Daily fluid gains and losses
>
> Each day the body gains and loses fluid through several different processes. The amounts shown below apply to adults; infants exchange a greater amount of fluid than adults.
>
> Gastric, intestinal, pancreatic, and biliary secretions total about 8,200 ml. However, because they're almost completely reabsorbed, they aren't usually counted in daily fluid gains and losses.
>
> **DAILY TOTAL INTAKE– 2,400 TO 3,200 ML**
> - Liquids–1,400 to 1,800 ml
> - Water in foods (solid)–700 to 1,000 ml
> - Water of oxidation (combined water and oxygen in the respiratory system)–300 to 400 ml
>
> **DAILY TOTAL OUTPUT– 2,400 TO 3,200 ML**
> - Lungs (respiration)–600 to 800 ml
> - Skin (perspiration)–300 to 500 ml
> - Kidneys (urine)–1,400 to 1,800 ml
> - Intestines (feces)–100 ml

The thirst mechanism also regulates water volume and interacts with hormones to maintain fluid balance. Thirst is experienced when water loss equals 2% of body weight or when osmolarity increases. Drinking water restores plasma volume and dilutes ECF osmolarity.

It's important to establish the patient's baseline fluid status before starting any fluid-replacement therapy. During I.V. therapy, changes in fluid status alert the nurse to impending fluid imbalances. (See *Identifying fluid imbalances*.)

Electrolytes

Electrolytes are a major component of body fluids. The six major electrolytes are:
- calcium
- chloride
- magnesium
- phosphorus
- potassium
- sodium.

As their name implies, electrolytes are associated with electricity. These vital substances are chemical compounds that dissociate in solution into electrically charged particles called ions. Like wiring for the body, the electrical charges of ions conduct current that's

Identifying fluid imbalances

By carefully assessing a patient before and during I.V. therapy, you can identify fluid imbalances early—before serious complications develop. The following assessment findings and test results indicate fluid deficit or excess.

FLUID DEFICIT
- Weight loss
- Increased, thready pulse rate
- Decreased blood pressure, commonly with orthostatic hypotension
- Decreased peripheral pulses
- Decreased central venous pressure
- Sunken eyes, dry conjunctivae, decreased tearing
- Poor skin turgor (not a reliable sign in elderly patients)
- Pale, cool skin
- Poor capillary refill (more than 2 seconds)
- Lack of moisture in groin and axillae
- Thirst
- Decreased salivation
- Dry mouth
- Dry, cracked lips
- Furrows in tongue
- Difficulty forming words (patient needs to moisten mouth first)
- Mental status changes
- Weakness
- Decreased urine output
- Increased hematocrit
- Increased electrolyte levels
- Increased blood urea nitrogen (BUN) levels
- Increased serum osmolarity
- Fever
- Increased specific gravity

FLUID EXCESS
- Weight gain
- Elevated blood pressure
- Bounding pulse that isn't easily obliterated
- Jugular vein distention
- Increased respiratory rate
- Dyspnea
- Moist crackles or rhonchi on auscultation
- Edema of dependent body parts; sacral edema in patients on bed rest; edema of feet and ankles in ambulatory patients
- Generalized edema
- Puffy eyelids
- Periorbital edema
- Slow emptying of hand veins when the arm is raised
- Decreased hematocrit
- Decreased electrolyte levels
- Decreased BUN levels
- Reduced serum osmolarity
- Increased central venous pressure
- Shallow respirations
- Skeletal muscle weakness
- Altered level of consciousness

necessary for normal cell function. (See *Understanding electrolytes*, pages 6 to 9.)

(Text continues on page 8.)

Understanding electrolytes

Six major electrolytes play important roles in maintaining chemical balance.

ELECTROLYTE AND NORMAL LEVEL	WHERE IT'S FOUND AND WHAT IT DOES
SODIUM (NA+) 135 to 145 mEq/L	• Major cation in extracellular fluid (ECF) • Maintains appropriate ECF osmolarity • Influences water distribution (with chloride) • Affects concentration, excretion, and absorption of potassium and chloride • Helps regulate acid-base balance • Aids nerve- and muscle-fiber impulse transmission
POTASSIUM (K+) 3.5 to 5.0 mEq/L	• Major cation in intracellular fluid (ICF) • Maintains cell electroneutrality • Maintains cell osmolarity • Assists in conduction of nerve impulses • Directly affects cardiac muscle contraction • Plays a major role in acid-base balance
CALCIUM (CA++) 8.9 to 10.1 mg/dl	• Major cation found in ECF of teeth and bones • Enhances bone strength and durability (along with phosphorus) • Helps maintain cell-membrane structure, function, and permeability • Affects activation, excitation, and contraction of cardiac and skeletal muscles • Participates in neurotransmitter release at synapses • Helps activate specific steps in blood coagulation • Activates serum complement in immune system function
CHLORIDE (CL-) 96 to 106 mEq/L	• Major anion found in ECF • Maintains serum osmolarity (along with Na^-) • Combines with major cations to create important compounds, such as sodium chloride (NaCl), hydrogen chloride (HCl), potassium chloride (KCl), and calcium chloride ($CaCl_2$)

IMBALANCES AND THEIR SIGNS AND SYMPTOMS

Hyponatremia: muscle weakness and twitching, decreased skin turgor, headache, tremor, seizures, coma
Hypernatremia: thirst, fever, flushed skin, oliguria, disorientation, dry, sticky membranes

Hypokalemia: decreased GI, skeletal muscle, and cardiac muscle function; decreased reflexes; rapid, weak, irregular pulse; muscle weakness or irritability; fatigue; decreased blood pressure; decreased bowel motility; paralytic ileus
Hyperkalemia: muscle weakness, nausea, diarrhea, oliguria, paresthesia (altered sensation) of the face, tongue, hands, and feet

Hypocalcemia: muscle tremor, muscle cramps, tetany, tonic–clonic seizures, paresthesia, bleeding, arrhythmias, hypotension, numbness or tingling in fingers, toes, and around the mouth
Hypercalcemia: lethargy, headache, muscle flaccidity, nausea, vomiting, anorexia, constipation, hypertension, polyuria

Hypochloremia: increased muscle excitability, tetany, decreased respirations
Hyperchloremia: stupor; rapid, deep breathing; muscle weakness

(continued)

Understanding electrolytes (continued)

ELECTROLYTE AND NORMAL LEVEL	WHERE IT'S FOUND AND WHAT IT DOES
PHOSPHORUS (P) 2.5 to 4.5 mg/dl	• Major anion found in ICF • Helps maintain bones and teeth • Helps maintain cell integrity • Plays a major role in acid-base balance (as a urinary buffer) • Promotes energy transfer to cells • Plays essential role in muscle, red blood cell, and neurologic function
MAGNESIUM (MG++) 1.5 to 2.5 mg/dl with 33% bound protein and remainder as free cations	• Major cation found in ICF (closely related to Ca++ and P) • Activates intracellular enzymes; active in carbohydrate and protein metabolism • Acts on myoneural vasodilation • Facilitates Na+ and K+ movement across all membranes • Influences Ca++ levels

FLUID AND ELECTROLYTE BALANCE

Fluids and electrolytes are usually discussed in tandem, especially where I.V. therapy is concerned, because fluid balance and electrolyte balance are interdependent. Any change in one alters the other, and any solution given I.V. can affect a patient's fluid and electrolyte balance.

Electrolyte balance

Not all electrolytes are distributed evenly. The major intracellular electrolytes are potassium and phosphorus. The major extracellular electrolytes are sodium and chloride.

ICF and ECF contain different electrolytes because the cell membranes separating the two compartments have selective permeability — that is, only certain ions can cross those membranes. Although ICF and ECF contain different solutes, the concentration levels of the two fluids are about equal when balance is maintained.

The two ECF components — ISF and intravascular fluid (plasma) — have identical electrolyte compositions. Pores in the capillary

IMBALANCES AND THEIR SIGNS AND SYMPTOMS

Hypophosphatemia: paresthesia (circumoral and peripheral), lethargy, speech defects (such as stuttering or stammering), muscle pain and tenderness
Hyperphosphatemia: renal failure, vague neuroexcitability to tetany and seizures, arrhythmias and muscle twitching with sudden rise in phosphate level

Hypomagnesemia: dizziness, confusion, seizures, tremor, leg and foot cramps, hyperirritability, arrhythmias, vasomotor changes, anorexia, nausea
Hypermagnesemia: drowsiness, lethargy, coma, arrhythmias, hypotension, vague neuromuscular changes (such as tremor), vague GI symptoms (such as nausea), peripheral vasodilation, facial flushing, sense of warmth, and a slow, weak pulse

---

walls allow electrolytes to move freely between the ISF and plasma, allowing for equal distribution of electrolytes in both substances.

However, the protein contents of ISF and plasma differ. ISF doesn't contain proteins because protein molecules are too large to pass through capillary walls. Plasma, on the other hand, has a high concentration of proteins.

Fluid movement: The regulating mechanism

Body fluids are in constant motion. Although separated by membranes, they continually move between the major fluid compartments. In addition to regulating fluid and electrolyte balance, this is how nutrients, waste products, and other substances get into and out of cells, organs, and body systems.

Fluid movement is influenced by membrane permeability and by colloid osmotic and hydrostatic pressures. Balance is maintained when solutes and fluids are distributed evenly on each side of the membrane. When this scale is tipped, solutes and fluids are able to restore balance by crossing membranes as needed.

Solutes and fluids have several modes for moving through membranes:
- diffusion (passive transport)
- active transport
- osmosis
- capillary filtration and reabsorption.

DIFFUSION
Most solutes move by diffusion — that is, they move from areas of higher concentration to areas of lower concentration. This change is referred to as "moving down the concentration gradient." The result is an equal distribution of solutes. Because energy isn't required, diffusion is considered a form of passive transport.

ACTIVE TRANSPORT
By contrast, in active transport, solutes move from areas of lower concentration to areas of higher concentration. This change, referred to as "moving against the concentration gradient," requires energy in the form of adenosine triphosphate.

In active transport, solutes are moved by physiologic pumps. You may be familiar with one active transport pump — the sodium-potassium pump. It moves sodium ions out of cells to the ECF and potassium ions into cells from the ECF. This balances sodium and potassium concentrations.

OSMOSIS
Fluids move by osmosis. Movement of water is caused by the existence of a concentration gradient. Water flows passively across the membrane, from an area of higher water concentration to an area of lower water concentration. This dilution process stops when the solute concentrations on both sides of the membrane are equal.

Osmosis between the ECF and ICF depends on the osmolarity (concentration) of the compartments. Normally, the osmotic (pulling) pressures of ECF and ICF balance one another.

Osmosis can create a fluid imbalance between the ECF and ICF compartments, despite equal concentrations of solute, if the concentrations aren't optimal. This can cause complications such as tissue edema.

CAPILLARY FILTRATION AND REABSORPTION
Of all the vessels in the vascular system, only capillaries have walls thin enough to let solutes pass. Water and solutes move across capillary walls by two opposing processes: filtration and reabsorption.

Filtration is the movement of substances from an area of high hydrostatic pressure to an area of lower hydrostatic pressure. (Hydrostatic pressure is the pressure on water at rest by the weight of water above it.) Capillary filtration forces fluid and solutes through capillary wall pores and into the ISF.

Unchecked, capillary filtration would cause plasma to move in only one direction—out of the capillaries. This movement would cause severe hypovolemia and shock.

Fortunately, capillary reabsorption keeps capillary filtration in check. During filtration, albumin (a protein that can't pass through capillary walls) remains behind in the diminishing volume of water. As the albumin concentration inside the capillaries increases, the albumin begins to draw water back in by osmosis. So, the water is reabsorbed by the capillaries.

The osmotic or pulling force of albumin in capillary reabsorption is called colloid osmotic pressure, or oncotic pressure. As long as capillary blood pressure exceeds colloid osmotic pressure, water and diffusible solutes can leave the capillaries and circulate into the ISF. When capillary blood pressure falls below colloid osmotic pressure, water and diffusible solutes return to the capillaries.

In any capillary, blood pressure normally exceeds colloid osmotic pressure up to the vessel's midpoint, and then falls below colloid osmotic pressure along the rest of the vessel. That's why capillary filtration takes place along the first half of a capillary and reabsorption occurs along the second half. As long as capillary blood pressure and plasma albumin levels remain normal, no change in the amount of water occurs.

Correcting imbalances

The effect an I.V. solution has on fluid compartments depends on how the solution's osmolarity compares with the patient's serum osmolarity.

Osmolarity is the concentration of a solution. It's expressed in milliosmols of solute per liter of solution (mOsm/L). Normally, serum has the same osmolarity as other body fluids, about 300 mOsm/L. A lower serum osmolarity suggests fluid overload; a higher serum osmolarity suggests hemoconcentration and dehydration.

When serum osmolarity increases or decreases, the physician may order I.V. solutions to maintain or restore fluid balance. There are three basic types of I.V. solutions:
- isotonic
- hypotonic
- hypertonic.

(See *Understanding osmolarity in I.V. solutions,* page 12.)

Understanding osmolarity in I.V. solutions

Solutions used for I.V. therapy may be isotonic, hypotonic, or hypertonic. The type you give a patient depends on whether you want to change or maintain his body fluid status.

ISOTONIC SOLUTION
An isotonic solution has an osmolarity about equal to that of serum. Because it stays in the intravascular space, it expands the intravascular compartment.

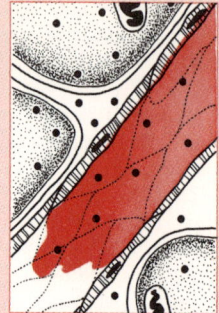

HYPOTONIC SOLUTION
A hypotonic solution has an osmolarity lower than that of serum. It shifts fluid out of the intravascular compartment, hydrating the cells and the interstitial compartments.

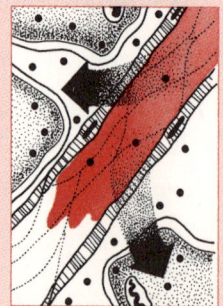

HYPERTONIC SOLUTION
A hypertonic solution has an osmolarity higher than that of serum. It draws fluid into the intravascular compartment from the cells and the interstitial compartments.

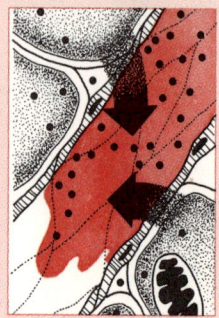

Isotonic solutions

An isotonic solution has the same osmolarity (or tonicity) as serum and other body fluids. Because the solution doesn't alter serum osmolarity, it stays where it's infused—inside the blood vessel (the intravascular compartment). The solution expands this compartment without pulling fluid from other compartments.

One indication for an isotonic solution is hypotension from hypovolemia. Common isotonic solutions include lactated Ringer's and normal saline.

Hypotonic solutions

A hypotonic solution has an osmolarity lower than serum osmolarity. When a patient receives a hypotonic solution, fluid shifts out of the blood vessels and into the cells and interstitial spaces, where osmolarity is higher. A hypotonic solution hydrates cells while reducing fluid in the circulatory system.

Hypotonic solutions may be ordered when diuretic therapy dehydrates cells. Other indications include hyperglycemic conditions, such as diabetic ketoacidosis and hyperosmolar hyperglycemic nonketotic syndrome. In these conditions, high serum glucose levels draw fluid out of cells. Examples of hypotonic solutions include half-normal saline, 0.33% sodium chloride, dextrose 2.5% in water, and dextrose 2.5%.

Because hypotonic solutions flood cells, certain patients shouldn't receive them. For example, patients with cerebral edema or increased intracranial pressure shouldn't receive hypotonic solutions because the increased ECF can cause further edema and tissue damage.

Hypertonic solutions

A hypertonic solution has an osmolarity higher than serum osmolarity. When a patient receives a hypertonic I.V. solution, serum osmolarity initially increases, causing fluid to be pulled from the interstitial and intracellular compartments into the blood vessels.

Hypertonic solutions may be ordered for patients postoperatively. That's because the shift of fluid into the blood vessels caused by a hypertonic solution has several beneficial effects for these patients. For example, the solution may:
- reduce the risk of edema
- stabilize blood pressure
- regulate urine output.

Quick guide to representative I.V. solutions

A solution is isotonic if its osmolarity falls within (or near) the normal range for serum (240 to 340 mOsm/L). A hypotonic solution has a lower osmolarity; a hypertonic solution, a higher osmolarity. This table lists common examples of the three types of I.V. solutions and provides key considerations for administering them.

OSMOLARITY TYPE	REPRESENTATIVES AND THEIR OSMOLARITIES
Isotonic	<ul><li>Lactated Ringer's (275 mOsm/L)</li><li>Ringer's (275 mOsm/L)</li><li>Normal saline (308 mOsm/L)</li><li>Dextrose 5% in water (D_5W) (260 mOsm/L)</li><li>5% albumin (308 mOsm/L)</li><li>Hetastarch (310 mOsm/L)</li></ul>
Hypotonic	<ul><li>Half-normal saline (154 mOsm/L)</li><li>0.33% sodium chloride (103 mOsm/L)</li><li>Dextrose 2.5% in water (126 mOsm/L)</li></ul>
Hypertonic	<ul><li>Dextrose 5% in half-normal saline (406 mOsm/L)</li><li>Dextrose 5% in normal saline (560 mOsm/L)</li><li>Dextrose 5% in lactated Ringer's (575 mOsm/L)</li><li>3% sodium chloride (1,025 mOsm/L)</li><li>25% albumin (1,500 mOsm/L)</li><li>7.5% sodium chloride (2,400 mOsm/L)</li></ul>

Some examples of hypertonic solutions are dextrose 5% in half-normal saline (405 mOsm/L), dextrose 5% in normal saline (560 mOsm/L), and dextrose 5% in lactated Ringer's (527 mOsm/L).

NURSING CONSIDERATIONS

- Because isotonic solutions expand the intravascular compartment, closely monitor the patient for signs of fluid overload, especially if he has hypertension or heart failure.
- Because the liver converts lactate to bicarbonate, don't give lactated Ringer's solution if the patient's blood pH exceeds 7.5.
- Don't give D_5W to a patient at risk for increased intracranial pressure (ICP) because it acts like a hypotonic solution. (Although usually considered isotonic, D_5W is actually isotonic only in the container. After administration, dextrose is quickly metabolized, leaving only water—a hypotonic fluid.)

- Administer cautiously. Hypotonic solutions cause a fluid shift from blood vessels into cells. This shift could cause cardiovascular collapse from intravascular fluid depletion and increased ICP from fluid shift into brain cells.
- Don't give hypotonic solutions to patients at risk for increased ICP from stroke, head trauma, or neurosurgery.
- Don't give hypotonic solutions to patients at risk for third-space fluid shifts (abnormal fluid shifts into the interstitial compartment or a body cavity)—for example, patients suffering from burns, trauma, or low serum protein levels from malnutrition or liver disease.

- Because hypertonic solutions greatly expand the intravascular compartment, administer them by I.V. pump and closely monitor the patient for circulatory overload.
- Hypertonic solutions pull fluid from the intracellular compartment, so don't give them to a patient with a condition that causes cellular dehydration—for example, diabetic ketoacidosis.
- Don't give hypertonic solutions to a patient with impaired heart or kidney function—his system can't handle the extra fluid.

Some common solutions are so representative of these types of solutions that they can be used to illustrate the role of I.V. therapy in restoring and maintaining fluid and electrolyte balance. (See *Quick guide to representative I.V. solutions.*)

TO ADMINISTER DRUGS
Giving drugs I.V. is rapid and effective. Commonly infused drugs include antibiotics, thrombolytics, histamine-receptor antagonists, antineoplastics, anticonvulsants, and cardiovascular drugs.

Drugs may be delivered long term by continuous infusion, over a short period, or directly as a single dose.

TO TRANSFUSE BLOOD AND BLOOD PRODUCTS
Your nursing responsibilities may include monitoring patients receiving transfusion therapy. Always know your state's nursing scope of practice guidelines regarding blood administration.

Blood products can be given through a peripheral or central I.V. line. Blood products are given for these reasons:
- to restore and maintain adequate blood volume
- to prevent cardiogenic shock
- to increase the blood's oxygen-carrying capacity
- to maintain hemostasis.

Whole blood is composed of plasma and these cellular elements:
- erythrocytes, or red blood cells
- leukocytes, or white blood cells
- thrombocytes, or platelets.

Each element is packaged separately for transfusion. Plasma may be delivered intact or separated into several components that can be given to correct various deficiencies. Whole blood transfusions are unnecessary unless the patient has lost massive quantities of blood in a short period.

TO DELIVER PARENTERAL NUTRIENTS AND NUTRITIONAL SUPPLEMENTS
Parenteral nutrition provides essential nutrients to the blood, organs, and cells by the I.V. route. It isn't the same as a five-course meal, but I.V. nutrients contain the essence of a balanced diet.

Solutions developed for total parenteral nutrition (TPN) provide all of these energy and nutrient requirements:
- proteins
- carbohydrates
- fats
- electrolytes
- vitamins
- trace elements
- water.

When your patient is receiving parenteral nutrition, keep close track of changes in his fluid and electrolyte status and glucose levels. You'll also need to collect data about your patient's response to the nutrient solution to detect early signs of complications, such as alterations in the pancreatic enzymes (lipase, amylase trypsin, and chymotrypsin) or in the albumin. A patient can receive TPN indefinitely.

Peripheral parenteral nutrition (PPN) is delivered by peripheral veins. PPN is used in limited nutritional therapy. The solution contains fewer nonprotein calories and lower amino acid concentrations than TPN solutions. It may also include lipid emulsions. It can be used to support the nutritional status of a patient who doesn't require total nutritional support. A patient can receive PPN for about 3 weeks.

Delivery routes and methods

I.V. solutions can be delivered using different routes into the body and using different methods. The routes and methods chosen depend on considerations described in this section.

ROUTES

Partly depending on an I.V. solution's concentration, administration may occur through one of two routes: a peripheral vein or a central vein. Usually, a low-concentration solution is infused through a peripheral vein in the arm or hand; a more concentrated solution must be given through a central vein. (See *Veins used in I.V. therapy,* page 18.)

METHODS

These are the three basic methods for delivering I.V. therapy:
- continuous infusion
- intermittent infusion
- direct injection.

Continuous infusion allows you to give a carefully regulated amount of fluid over a prolonged period. For intermittent infusion, a solution (commonly a drug) is given for shorter periods at set intervals. Direct injection (sometimes called I.V. push) is used to deliver a single dose (bolus) of a drug.

The choice of I.V. delivery method depends not only on the purpose and duration of therapy but also on the patient's condition, age, and health history.

Veins used in I.V. therapy

This illustration shows the veins commonly used for peripheral and central venous therapy.

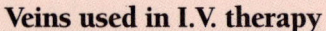

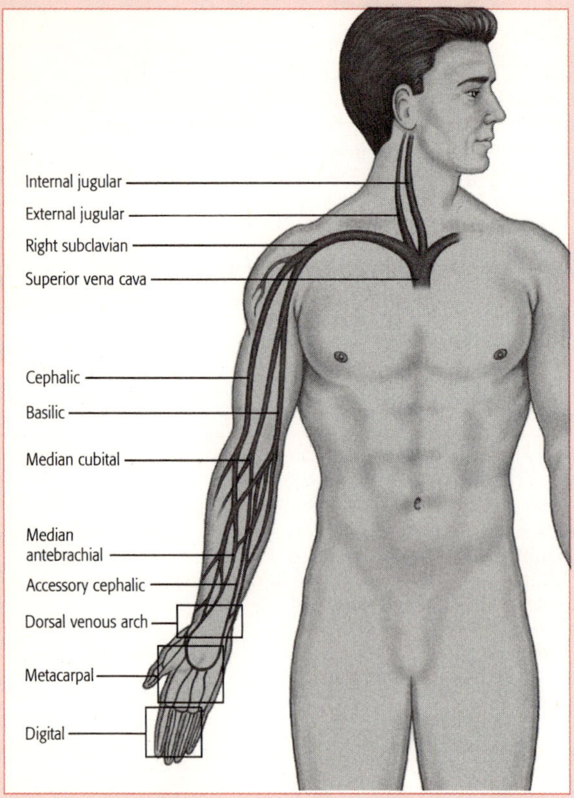

- Internal jugular
- External jugular
- Right subclavian
- Superior vena cava
- Cephalic
- Basilic
- Median cubital
- Median antebrachial
- Accessory cephalic
- Dorsal venous arch
- Metacarpal
- Digital

At times, a patient may receive I.V. therapy by more than one delivery method. Also, variations of each delivery method may be used. Some therapies also require extra equipment. For example, in some long-term chemotherapy, an implanted central venous access device is needed. (See *Comparing I.V. delivery methods.*)

Comparing I.V. delivery methods

This table lists the indications, advantages, and disadvantages of methods commonly used to administer I.V. medications.

METHOD AND INDICATIONS	ADVANTAGES	DISADVANTAGES
CONTINUOUS INFUSION		
Through primary line • When continuous serum levels are needed • When consistent fluid levels are needed	• Maintains steady serum levels • Lowers the risk of rapid shock and vein irritation from a large volume of fluid diluting the drug	• Increases the risk of incompatibility with drugs administered by piggyback infusion • Restricts patient mobility when the patient is connected to an I.V. system • Increases the risk of undetected infiltration because slow infusion makes it difficult to see swelling in the area of infiltration
Through secondary line, which is connected to a primary line • When the patient requires continuous infusion of two or more compatible admixtures administered at different rates • When there's a moderate to high chance of abruptly stopping one admixture without infusing the drug remaining in the I.V. tubing	• Permits the primary infusion and each secondary infusion to be given at different rates • Permits the primary line to be shut off and kept standing by to maintain venous access in case a secondary line must be abruptly stopped	• Eliminates the use of drugs with immediate incompatibility • Increases the risk of phlebitis or vein irritation from an increased number of drugs • Uses multiple I.V. systems (for example, primary lines with secondary lines attached), which can create physical barriers to patient care and limit patient mobility, especially those with electronic pumps or controllers

(continued)

Continuous infusion

A continuous infusion helps maintain a constant therapeutic drug level. It's also used to provide I.V. fluid therapy or parenteral nutrition.

Comparing I.V. delivery methods (continued)

METHOD AND INDICATIONS	ADVANTAGES	DISADVANTAGES
INTERMITTENT INFUSION		
Piggyback method, which requires connecting a second administration set to a primary line ● Commonly used with drugs given over short periods at varying intervals (for example, antibiotics and gastric secretion inhibitors)	● Avoids multiple intramuscular injections ● Permits repeated administration of drugs through a single I.V. line ● Provides high drug blood levels for short periods	● May cause periods when the drug level becomes too low to be clinically effective (for example, when peak and trough times aren't considered in the medication order)
Saline lock, which allows for maintenance of venous access ● When the patient requires constant venous access but not continuous infusion	● Provides venous access for patients with fluid restrictions ● Allows better patient mobility between doses ● Preserves veins by reducing frequent venipuncture ● Lowers cost	● Requires close monitoring during administration so the device can be flushed on completion ● Most commonly used in adults with peripheral I.V. access devices
Volume-control set, which has a medication chamber that allows it to deliver small doses over an extended period ● When the patient requires a low volume of fluid	● Requires only one large-volume container and prevents fluid overload from runaway infusion	● May have high equipment costs ● Carries a high contamination risk ● Requires that the flow clamp be closed when the set empties, if set doesn't contain a membrane that blocks the air passage when it's empty

Continuous infusion has advantages. Less time is spent mixing solutions and hanging containers than with the intermittent method. You'll also handle less tubing and access the patient's I.V. device less often, decreasing the risk of infection.

Comparing I.V. delivery methods *(continued)*

METHOD AND INDICATIONS	ADVANTAGES	DISADVANTAGES
DIRECT INJECTION		
Into a vein, which generally doesn't involve an administration set and is commonly referred to as *I.V. push* ● When a nonirritating drug with a low risk of immediate adverse reactions is required for a patient with no other I.V. needs (for example, single injection of furosemide, a diuretic)	● Eliminates the risk of complications from an implanted (indwelling) venous access device ● Eliminates the inconvenience of an indwelling venous access device	● Can only be given by a physician or specially certified nurse ● Requires venipuncture, which can cause patient anxiety ● Requires two syringes—one to administer the medication and one to flush the vein after administration ● Requires dilution of the medication before injection ● Risks infiltration (puncture of the vein, allowing the solution to enter the surrounding tissue) from the steel needle ● Makes it impossible to dilute the drug or interrupt delivery when irritation occurs
Through an existing infusion line ● When the patient requires immediate high blood levels of a medication (for example, regular insulin, dextrose 50%, atropine, or antihistamines) ● In emergencies, when the drug must be given quickly for immediate effect	● Doesn't require time or authorization to perform venipuncture because the vein is already accessed ● Doesn't require needle puncture, which can cause patient anxiety ● Allows the use of an I.V. solution to test the patency of the venous access device before drug administration ● Allows continued venous access in case of adverse reactions	● Carries the same inconveniences and complication risks as an indwelling venous access device

Continuous infusion has some disadvantages, too. The patient may become distressed if the equipment hinders mobility and interferes with other activities of daily living. Also, the drip rate must be carefully monitored to ensure that the I.V. fluid or drug doesn't infuse too rapidly or too slowly.

Intermittent infusion

The most common and flexible method of giving I.V. drugs is by intermittent infusion. In intermittent infusion, drugs are given over a specified period at varying intervals, maintaining therapeutic levels. A small volume (1 to 250 ml) may be delivered over several minutes or a few hours, depending on the order. You can deliver an intermittent infusion through a primary line (the most common method) or a secondary line. The secondary line is usually connected or piggybacked into the primary line by way of a Y-site (a Y-shaped section of tubing with a self-sealing access port).

Direct injection

You might say that I.V. therapy by direct injection gets right to the point. A vein can be accessed directly for a single dose of a prescribed drug or solution. The needle is then removed when the bolus is completed. A bolus injection may also be given through an intermittent infusion device that's already in place.

Infusion rates

A key aspect of administering I.V. therapy is maintaining accurate infusion rates for the solutions. If an infusion runs too fast or too slow, your patient may suffer complications, such as phlebitis, infiltration, circulatory overload (possibly leading to heart failure and pulmonary edema), and adverse drug reactions. Volume-control devices and the correct administration set help prevent such complications.

ADMINISTRATION SETS

You need to choose the correct administration set for your patient's infusion. Your choice depends on the type of infusion to be provided, the type of infusion container, and the need for a volume-control device.

I.V. administration sets come in two forms: vented and unvented. The vented set is for containers that have no venting system (I.V.

plastic bags and some bottles). The unvented are for those bottles that have their own venting system.

I.V. administration sets come with various other features as well, including ports for infusing secondary drugs and filters for blocking microbes, irritants, or large particles. The tubing also varies. Some types are designed to enhance the proper functioning of devices that help regulate the flow rate. Other tubing is used specifically for continuous or intermittent infusion or for infusing parenteral nutrition and blood.

Rates and sets
There are two basic types of infusion rates available with I.V. administration sets: macrodrip and microdrip.

Each set delivers a specific number of drops per milliliter (gtt/ml). Macrodrip delivers 10, 15, or 20 gtt/ml; microdrip delivers 60 gtt/ml. Regardless of the type of set you use, the formula for calculating infusion rates is the same. (See *Calculating infusion rates,* page 24.)

REGULATING INFUSION RATES
When a patient's condition requires you to maintain precise I.V. infusion rates, use one of these infusion control devices:
- clamps
- volumetric pumps
- rate minders.

When you regulate I.V. infusion rate with a clamp, the rate is usually measured in drops per minute (gtt/minute). If you use a pump, the infusion rate is measured in milliliters per hour (ml/hour).

I.V. clamps
You can regulate the infusion rate with two types of clamps: screw and roller. The screw clamp offers greater accuracy, but the roller clamp, used for standard fluid therapy, is faster and easier to manipulate. A third type, the slide clamp, can stop or start the infusion but can't regulate the rate.

Pumps
New pumps are being developed all the time; be sure to attend instruction sessions to learn how to use them. On your unit, keep a file of instruction manuals (provided by the manufacturers) for each piece of equipment used.

24 ■ Introduction to I.V. therapy

BEST PRACTICE

Calculating infusion rates

When calculating the infusion rate (drops per minute) of I.V. solutions, remember that the number of drops required to deliver 1 ml varies with the type of administration set used and its manufacturer:
- Administration sets are of two types—macrodrip (the standard type) and microdrip. Macrodrip delivers 10, 15, or 20 gtt/ml; microdrip usually delivers 60 gtt/ml (see illustrations).
- Manufacturers calibrate their devices differently, so be sure to look for the "drop factor"—expressed in drops per milliliter, or gtt/ml—in the packaging that accompanies the set you're using. (This packaging also has crucial information about such things as special infusions and blood transfusions.)

When you know your device's drop factor, use the following formula to calculate specific flow rates:

$$\frac{\text{volume of infusion (in milliliters)}}{\text{time of infusion (in minutes)}} \times$$

drop factor (in drops per milliliter) =

infusion rate (in drops per minute)

After you calculate the infusion rate for the set you're using, remove your watch or position your wrist so you can look at your watch and the drops at the same time. Next, adjust the clamp to achieve the ordered infusion rate and count the drops for 1 full minute. Readjust the clamp as necessary and count the drops for another minute. Continue adjusting the clamp and counting the drops until you have the correct rate.

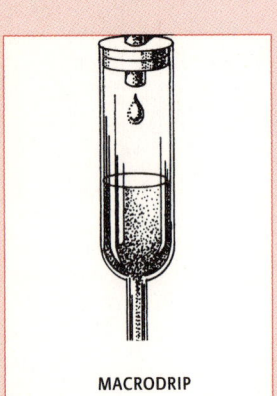

MACRODRIP

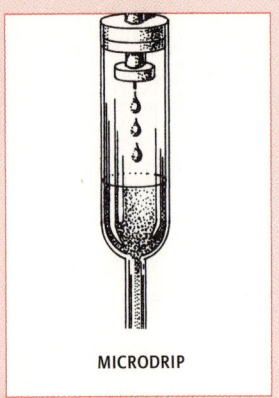

MICRODRIP

BEST PRACTICE

Using a time tape

Here's a simple way to monitor I.V. infusion rate: Attach a piece of tape or a preprinted strip to the I.V. container; then write hourly times on the tape or strip beginning with the time you hung the solution.

By comparing the actual time with the label time, you can quickly see if the rate needs to be adjusted. Remember that you should never increase I.V. rates unless you first check with the physician.

Rate minder

Another type of infusion control device is the rate minder, which resembles a roller clamp. This device is added to the I.V. tubing. By setting the rate minder to the desired flow rate, you adjust the clamp to deliver that rate. Be sure to label the infusion bag with the rate in milliliters per hour.

Rate minders have some limitations. Because the infusion rate may vary by as much as 5%, the infusion must be checked frequently to prevent a too-rapid, too-slow, or nonflowing infusion. The other drawback is that the rate minders usually don't deliver infusions at rates lower than 5 to 10 ml/hour. For this reason, they're used mainly for adult patients and only with noncritical infusions.

When you're using a clamp for infusion regulation, you must monitor the infusion rate closely and adjust as needed. Such factors as vein spasm, vein pressure changes, patient movement, manipulations of the clamp, and bent or kinked tubing can cause the rate to vary markedly. For easy monitoring, use a time tape, which marks the prescribed solution level at hourly intervals. (See *Using a time tape.*)

Other factors that affect infusion rate include the type of I.V. fluid and its viscosity, the height of the infusion container, the type of administration set, and the size and position of the venous access device.

CHECKING INFUSION RATES

Infusion rates can be fickle; they need to be checked and adjusted regularly. The frequency at which infusion rates are checked depends on the patient's condition, age, and the solution or medication being administered.

Many nurses check the I.V. infusion rate every time they're in a patient's room and after each position change. The infusion rate should be assessed more frequently for some patients, such as:
- critically ill patients
- patients with conditions that might be exacerbated by fluid overload
- pediatric patients
- elderly patients
- patients receiving a drug that can cause tissue damage if infiltration occurs.

If the infusion rate slows significantly, you can usually get it back on schedule by adjusting the rate slightly. Don't make a major adjustment, though. If the rate must be increased by more than 30%, check with the physician.

You should also time an infusion control device or rate minder for 1 to 2 hours per shift. (These devices have an error rate ranging from 2% to 10%.) Before using any infusion control device, become thoroughly familiar with its features. Attend instruction sessions and practice using the equipment for the instructor until you learn the system.

Professional and legal standards

As a nurse, you have a legal and ethical responsibility to your patients. The good news is that if you honor these duties and meet the appropriate standards of care, you will be prepared for court. You can also help by being familiar with all of the information in the physician's orders and being able to recognize incomplete or incorrectly written orders for I.V. therapy. (See *Reading an I.V. order.*)

By becoming aware of professional standards and laws related to giving I.V. therapy, you can provide the best care for your patients and protect yourself legally. Professional and legal standards are defined by state nurse practice acts, federal regulations, and facility policies.

Administering drugs and solutions to patients is one of the most legally perilous tasks nurses perform. A 1995 study in Missouri reported a high incidence of errors with I.V. solution administration, such as the use of incorrect solutions or solutions administered by an incorrect route.

Unfortunately, the number of lawsuits directed against nurses who are involved in I.V. therapy is increasing. Many lawsuits center on errors in infusion pump use. Lawsuits may also result from ad-

> ### Reading an I.V. order
>
> Orders for I.V. therapy may be standardized for different illnesses and therapies (such as burn treatment) or individualized for a particular patient. Some facility policies dictate an automatic stop order for I.V. fluids. For example, I.V. orders are good for 24 hours from the time they're written, unless otherwise specified.
>
> **IT'S COMPLETE**
> A complete order for I.V. therapy should specify:
> - type and amount of solution
> - any additives and their concentrations (such as 10 mEq potassium chloride in 500 ml dextrose 5% in water)
> - rate and volume of infusion
> - duration of infusion.
>
> **WHEN IT ISN'T COMPLETE**
> If you find that an order isn't complete or if you think an I.V. order is inappropriate because of the patient's condition, consult with the physician.

ministration of the wrong drug dosage, inappropriate placement of an I.V. line, and failure to monitor for adverse reactions, infiltration, dislodged I.V. equipment, or other problems.

COURT CASES

The following are examples of lawsuits involving I.V. therapy.

In Los Angeles, a nurse administered midazolam (Versed) to an infant through a port in an I.V. line, which led to the infant's death. This nurse had never administered I.V. Versed to an infant or child before. A facility protocol prohibited the use of Versed on the pediatric floor. The manufacturer recommended a dosage of 0.1 mg/kg, and the infant weighed 20 lb (9 kg). The hospital record indicated 5 mg had been administered. The parents were awarded $225,000 in a settlement.

In another case, continuous infusion of 145 mg of morphine over 18 hours led to a patient's death. The physician failed to limit the amount to be infused. Nevertheless, the charge nurse and staff nurse were held accountable for failing to recognize a "gross overdose." The patient's widow and children were awarded over $2 million for lost wages and general damages.

In Illinois, a nurse administered the wrong dose of lidocaine (Xylocaine). The order was for 100 mg; the nurse injected 2 g. The packaging caused confusion: the Xylocaine was provided in a 2-g syringe for mixing into an I.V. solution and in a 100-mg syringe for direct injection. The nurse accidentally used the 2-g syringe. However, information about previous overdose incidents from the Food and Drug Administration and medical literature had been available to the hospital.

In Ohio, a nurse failed to clamp a pump regulating the flow of an antibiotic to a child through a central line. This resulted in delivery of nearly seven times the prescribed dosage of gentamicin, causing the child to become totally deaf.

In Pennsylvania, an emergency department nurse misplaced an I.V. line, which infiltrated the patient's hand, resulting in reflex sympathetic dystrophy. The patient couldn't return to work and won a $702,000 award.

Several other lawsuits have involved allegations that a nurse struck a patient's radial nerve during insertion of an I.V. line. Such injuries can cause compartment syndrome and may require emergency fasciotomy, skin grafts, and other surgery. Uncorrected compartment syndrome can progress to gangrene and amputation of fingers. One New York case involving finger amputation resulted in a $40 million jury verdict, which was later reduced to $5 million.

When monitoring an I.V. line, listening to the patient is as important as monitoring the site, pump, and tubing. In the Tampa, Florida, case of *Frank v. Hillsborough County Hospital*, a patient's frequent complaints of pain were ignored. The patient suffered permanent nerve damage and later obtained an award of almost $60,000.

STATE NURSE PRACTICE ACTS

Each state has a nurse practice act that broadly defines the legal scope of nursing practice. Your state's nurse practice act is the most important law affecting your work.

Every nurse is expected to care for patients within defined limits. If a nurse gives care beyond those limits, she becomes vulnerable to charges of violating her state's nurse practice act. For a copy of your state's nurse practice act, contact your state's nurse's association or board of nursing.

Many state nurse practice acts do address whether licensed practical nurses (LPNs) or licensed vocational nurses (LVNs) can administer I.V. therapy. This is important for LPNs and LVNs as well as for the registered nurses who are supervising or training them.

FEDERAL REGULATIONS

The federal government issues regulations and establishes policies related to I.V. therapy administration. For example, it mandates adherence to standards of I.V. therapy practice for health care facilities so they can be eligible to receive reimbursement under Medicare, Medicaid, and other programs.

Medicare and Medicaid, the two major federal health care programs, serve about 75 million Americans. They're run by the Centers for Medicare and Medicaid Services (CMS), part of the Department of Health and Human Services. The office formulates national Medicare policy, including policies related to I.V. therapy, but contracts with private insurance companies to oversee claims and make payment for services and supplies provided under Medicare. These agencies, in turn, enforce Medicare and Medicaid policy by accepting or denying claims for reimbursement. When reviewing claims, agencies may evaluate practices and quality of care — an important factor underlying the emphasis on proper documentation in health care.

Medicaid, which serves certain low-income people, is a state and federal partnership administered by a state agency. There are broad federal requirements for Medicaid, but states have a wide degree of flexibility to design their own programs.

To be eligible for reimbursement, health care agencies must comply with the standards of a complex network of regulators. Consider, for example, a patient receiving I.V. drugs at home with a reusable pump. This patient is primarily covered by Medicare, with secondary Medicaid coverage. A variety of carriers, fiscal intermediaries, and agencies share responsibility for reimbursement and regulatory oversight of the patient's care:

- An insurance carrier contracts with Medicare to cover such services as refilling the pump.
- A separate insurance carrier (a durable medical equipment carrier designated by CMS) covers administered drugs, the pump, and pump supplies.
- Another insurance carrier (called a fiscal intermediary) contracts with Medicare to cover preliminary in-hospital training of the patient in I.V. therapy techniques.
- A Medicaid agency also covers a portion of the patient's care.

Nursing documentation must be complete to meet the requirements of all these different agencies. The underlying (although unstated) philosophy of these agencies is that "if it isn't documented, it isn't done." The regulatory network is becoming more complicated as many Medicare and Medicaid patients are being covered by managed care organizations that have their own rules and procedures.

FACILITY POLICY

Every health care facility has I.V. therapy policies for nurses. Such policies are required to obtain accreditation from the Joint Commission on Accreditation of Healthcare Organizations (JCAHO) and other accrediting bodies. These policies can't go beyond what a state's nurse practice act permits, but they more specifically define your duties and responsibilities.

Awareness of facility policy is particularly important in rapidly developing areas of practice such as home care where the intensity of service and patient needs are increasing dramatically. For example, home health nurses need to be acutely aware of patient- and family-education policies because infusion systems are being used in the home 24 hours per day without the presence of full-time nursing staff.

The Infusion Nurses Society (INS) has developed a set of standards, the *Infusion Nursing Standards of Practice,* that are commonly used by committees developing facility policy. According to the INS, the goals of these standards are to "protect and preserve the patient's right to safe, quality care and protect the nurse who administers infusion therapy." These standards address all aspects of I.V. nursing. For more information, contact the INS at (781) 440-9408 or at *www.ins1.org.*

Documentation

You need to document I.V. therapy for several reasons. Proper documentation provides:
- an accurate description of care that can serve as legal protection (for example, as evidence that a prescribed treatment was administered)
- a mechanism for recording and retrieving information
- a record for health care insurers of equipment and supplies used.

(See *Documenting I.V. therapy*.)

TYPES OF FORMS

I.V. therapy may be documented using progress notes, a sequential system, a special I.V. therapy sheet or flow sheet, a nursing plan of care on the patient's chart, or an intake and output sheet.

In addition to documentation in the patient's chart, you need to label the dressing on the catheter insertion site. Whenever you change the dressing, label the new one. (See *How to label a dressing,* page 32.)

You should also label the fluid container and place a time tape on it. With a child, you may need to label the volume-control set as well. In labeling the container and the set, follow your facility's policy and procedures. (See *How to label an I.V. bag,* page 33.)

> **DOCUMENTATION TIPS**
>
> ## Documenting I.V. therapy
>
> When documenting I.V. therapy, keep these points in mind.
>
> ### STARTING I.V. THERAPY
> When documenting the insertion of a venous access device or the beginning of therapy, specify:
> - size and type of the device
> - name of the person who inserted the device
> - date and time
> - site location
> - type of solution
> - any additives
> - infusion rate
> - use of an electronic infusion device or other type of flow controller
> - complications, patient response, and nursing interventions
> - patient teaching and evidence of patient understanding (for example, ability to explain instructions or perform a return demonstration)
> - number of attempts (both successful and unsuccessful).
>
> ### MAINTAINING I.V. THERAPY
> When documenting I.V. therapy maintenance, specify:
> - condition of the site
> - site care provided
> - dressing changes
> - site changes
> - tubing and solution changes
> - your teaching and evidence of patient understanding.
>
> ### STOPPING I.V. THERAPY
> When you document the discontinuation of I.V. therapy, be sure to specify:
> - time and date
> - reason for discontinuing therapy
> - assessment of venipuncture site before and after the venous access device is removed
> - complications, patient reactions, and nursing interventions
> - integrity of the venous access device on removal
> - follow-up actions (such as applying a bandage to the site or restarting the I.V. infusion in another extremity).

Sequential system

One way to document I.V. solutions throughout therapy is to number each container sequentially. For example, if a patient is to receive normal saline solution at 125 ml/hour (3,000 ml/day) on day 1, number the 1,000-ml containers as 1, 2, and 3. If another 3,000 ml is ordered on day 2, number those containers as 4, 5, and 6. This system may reduce administration errors. Also, check your facility's policy and procedures; some facilities require beginning the count again if the type of fluid changes, while others keep the count sequential regardless of the type of fluid.

> **Best practice**
>
> ## How to label a dressing
>
> To label a new dressing over an I.V. site, include:
> - date of insertion
> - gauge and length of venipuncture device
> - date and time of the dressing change
> - your initials.

Flow sheets

Flow sheets highlight specific patient information with established aspects of nursing care. They have spaces for recording dates, times, and specific interventions. When you use an I.V. flow sheet, record these items:

- date
- flow rate
- use of an electronic flow device or flow controller
- type of solution
- sequential solution container
- date and time of dressing and tubing changes.

Intake and output sheets

When you're documenting I.V. therapy on an intake and output sheet, follow these guidelines:

- If the patient is a child, note fluid levels on the I.V. containers hourly. If the patient is an adult, note these levels at least twice per shift.
- With children and intensive care patients, record intake of all I.V. infusions, including fluids, drugs, flush solutions, and blood and blood products, every 1 to 2 hours.
- Document the total amount of each infusion and totals of all infusions at least every shift, so you can monitor fluid balance.
- Note output hourly or less often (but at least once each shift), depending on the patient's condition. Output includes urine, stool, vomitus, and gastric drainage. For an acutely ill or unstable patient, you may need to assess urine output every 15 minutes.
- Read fluid levels from the containers or electronic volume-control device to estimate the amounts infused and the amounts remaining to be infused.

> **BEST PRACTICE**
>
> ### How to label an I.V. bag
>
> To properly label an I.V. solution container, include (in addition to the time tape):
> - patient's name, identification number, and room number
> - date and time the container was hung
> - any additives and their amounts
> - rate at which the solution is to run
> - sequential container number
> - expiration date and time of infusion
> - your name.
>
> When you place the label on the bag, make sure you don't cover up the name of the I.V. solution.

Patient teaching

Although you may be accustomed to I.V. therapy, many patients aren't. Your patient may be apprehensive about the procedure and concerned that his condition has worsened.

Teaching the patient and, when appropriate, members of his family will help him relax and take the mystery out of I.V. therapy. Begin by determining your patient's previous infusion experience, his expectations, and his knowledge of venipuncture and I.V. therapy. Base the teaching on your findings.

Your teaching should include these steps:
- Describe the procedure. Tell the patient that "I.V." means "inside the vein" and that a plastic catheter or needle will be placed in his vein.
- Explain that fluids containing certain nutrients or drugs will flow from a bag or bottle through a length of tubing, and then through the catheter or needle into his vein.
- Tell the patient how long the catheter or needle may stay in place, and explain that his physician will decide how much and what type of fluid and drugs he needs.
- Give the patient as much information as possible. Consider providing pamphlets, sample catheters and I.V. equipment, slides, videotapes, and other appropriate information. Make sure you tell the whole story.

- Tell the patient that although he may feel pain briefly as the needle goes in, the discomfort will stop when the catheter or needle is in place.
- Explain why I.V. therapy is needed and how the patient can help by holding still and not withdrawing if he feels pain when the needle is inserted.
- Explain that the I.V. fluids may feel cold at first, but the sensation should last only a few minutes.
- Instruct the patient to report any discomfort he feels after therapy begins.
- Explain activity restrictions such as those related to bathing and moving about.
- Give the patient time to express his concerns and fears, and take the time to provide reassurance. Encourage him to use stress-reduction techniques such as deep, slow breathing. Allow him and his family to participate in his care as much as possible.
- Make sure you evaluate how well your patient and members of the patient's family understand your instruction. Evaluate their understanding while you're teaching and when you're done. You can do this by asking frequent questions and having them explain or demonstrate what you have taught.
- Document your teaching in the patient's records. Note what you taught and how well the patient understood it.

2

PERIPHERAL I.V. THERAPY

Few nursing responsibilities require more time, knowledge, and skill than administering peripheral I.V. therapy. At the bedside, you need to assemble the equipment, prepare the patient, insert the venous access device, regulate the I.V. flow rate, and monitor the patient for possible adverse effects. You also have other responsibilities, such as checking the physician's orders, ordering and preparing supplies and equipment, labeling solutions and tubing, and documenting your nursing interventions. (See *Documenting I.V. insertion*.)

DOCUMENTATION TIPS

Documenting I.V. insertion

When you start an I.V. line, be sure to document the following information in all areas required by your facility's policy, such as the patient care Kardex, intake and output flow sheets, patient chart, and medication sheets.

- Date and time of the venipuncture
- Number of the solution container (if required by facility policy and procedures)
- Type and amount of solution
- Name and dosage of additives in the solution
- Type of infusion device used, including length and gauge
- Venipuncture site
- Number of insertion attempts, if more than one
- Infusion rate
- Adverse reactions and the actions taken to correct them
- Patient teaching and evidence of patient understanding
- Name of the person initiating the infusion

Perhaps the most challenging aspect of peripheral I.V. therapy is performing the venipuncture itself. You need good hands and a sharp eye, plus lots of practice — it's worth the effort, both in terms of positive outcome and patient satisfaction. As you gain experience, you'll learn to perform even difficult venipunctures confidently and successfully.

BASICS OF PERIPHERAL I.V. THERAPY

Peripheral I.V. therapy is ordered whenever venous access is needed, when a patient requires surgery, transfusion therapy, or emergency care. It's also used to maintain hydration, restore fluid and electrolyte balance, provide fluids for resuscitation, or administer I.V. drugs, blood and blood components, and nutrients for metabolic support.

Peripheral I.V. therapy offers easy access to veins and rapid administration of solutions, blood, and drugs. It allows continuous administration of drugs to produce rapid systemic changes. It's also easy to monitor.

Peripheral I.V. therapy is an invasive procedure that carries risks, such as bleeding, infiltration, and infection. Rapid infusion of some drugs can produce hearing loss, bone marrow depression, kidney or heart damage, and other irreversible adverse effects. Finally, peripheral I.V. therapy can't be used indefinitely and costs more than oral, subcutaneous, or I.M. drug therapy.

Despite its risks, peripheral I.V. therapy remains at the heart of modern medicine and is a crucial contribution that nurses make to their patients' well-being. The key is to do it well, and that starts with preparation.

Preparing for venipuncture and infusion

Before performing a venipuncture, talk with the patient, select and prepare the proper equipment, and choose the best access site and venipuncture device.

PREPARING THE PATIENT

Before approaching the patient, check his medical record for allergies and his disease history for the diagnosis and care plan. Review the physician's orders, noting pertinent laboratory results that might affect the administration or outcome of the prescribed therapy.

Many patients will be apprehensive. Among other things, this anxiety may cause vasoconstriction, making the venipuncture more

> ## Teaching a patient about peripheral I.V. therapy
>
> Many patients feel apprehensive about peripheral I.V. therapy. Before you begin therapy, teach the patient what to expect before, during, and after the procedure. Thorough patient teaching can reduce his anxiety, making therapy easier. Follow the guidelines below.
>
> ### DESCRIBE THE PROCEDURE
> - Tell the patient that "intravenous" means "inside the vein" and that a plastic catheter (plastic tube) or needle will be placed in his vein. Explain that fluids containing certain nutrients or drugs will flow from an I.V. bag or bottle through a length of tubing, and then through the plastic catheter or needle into his vein.
> - If you know about how long the catheter or needle will stay in place, tell the patient. Explain that the physician will decide how much and what type of fluid he needs.
> - Mention that he may feel some pain during insertion but that the discomfort will stop once the catheter or needle is in place.
> - Tell him that the I.V. fluid may feel cold at first, but this sensation should last only a few minutes.
> - Explain that removing a peripheral I.V. line is a simple procedure. Tell the patient that pressure will be applied to the site until the bleeding stops. Reassure him that, once the device is out and the bleeding stops, he'll be able to use his arm as usual.
>
> ### CAUTIONS
> - Tell the patient to report any discomfort after the catheter or needle has been inserted and the fluid has begun to flow.
> - Explain any restrictions. If appropriate, tell the patient that he can walk while receiving therapy. Depending on the insertion site and the device, he may also be able to shower or take a tub bath during therapy.
> - Teach the patient how to assist in I.V. system care. Tell him not to pull at the insertion site or tubing and not to remove the container from the I.V. pole. Also, tell him not to kink the tubing or lie on it. Explain that he should call a nurse if the infusion rate suddenly slows down or speeds up.

difficult for you and more painful for the patient. Careful patient teaching and a confident, understanding attitude will help your patient relax and cooperate during the procedure. (See *Teaching a patient about peripheral I.V. therapy*.)

After you complete your teaching, give your patient privacy by asking visitors to leave and drawing the curtains around the bed if another patient is in the room. Have him put on a gown if he isn't already wearing one, and remove any jewelry from the arm where the I.V. will be inserted. When the patient is ready, position him comfortably in the bed, preferably on his back. Make sure that the area is well lit and the bed is in a position that allows you to maneuver easily when inserting the infusion device.

SELECTING THE EQUIPMENT

Besides the venipuncture device, peripheral I.V. therapy requires a solution container, an administration set (usually with an in-line filtration system), and an infusion pump or controller (if needed).

Solution containers

Most health care facilities use plastic bags for the routine administration of I.V. fluids. Glass must be used to deliver drugs that are absorbed by plastic (such as nitroglycerin) and for albumin and immune globulin preparations.

PLASTIC

Because they're available in soft, flexible bags or semirigid rectangular containers, plastic solution containers allow easy storage, transportation, and disposal. Unlike glass bottles, they collapse as fluid flows out and don't require air venting, thus reducing the risk of air embolism or airborne contamination. In addition, plastic containers aren't likely to break, but can easily be punctured.

GLASS

In contrast, glass containers don't collapse as fluid flows out and require vented tubing. A vented I.V. administration set has an extra-filtered port near the spike that allows air to enter and displace fluid. This helps the solution flow correctly.

In addition, the glass system's crystal-clear transparency allows for better visualization of contents and more accurate reading of fluid level.

Administration sets

There are three major types of I.V. administration sets:
- basic, or *primary*
- add-a-line, or *secondary line*
- volume-control.

Each type has a drip chamber that may be vented or nonvented (glass containers require venting; plastic ones don't) and a drip system: macrodrip or microdrip. (See *Comparing I.V. administration sets,* pages 40 and 41.)

A macrodrip system delivers a solution in large quantities at rapid rates. A microdrip system delivers a smaller amount of solution with each drop and is used for children or adults who need small or closely regulated amounts of I.V. solution.

Selecting the correct set requires knowing the type of solution container being used and comparing the set's infusion rate with the nature of the I.V. solution — the more viscous the solution, the larger the drops and, so, the fewer drops per milliliter. Also, make sure that the intended solution can be infused using a filtration system; otherwise, you'll need an infusion set without the filtration component.

Depending on the type of therapy ordered, you may need to supplement the administration set with other equipment, such as stopcocks, extension loops, and needleless systems.

BASIC I.V. SETS
Basic I.V. administration sets range from 70″ to 110″ (178 to 279 cm) long. They're used to deliver any I.V. solution or to infuse solutions through an intermittent infusion device. A Y-site provides a secondary injection port for a separate or simultaneous infusion of two compatible solutions. A macrodrip set generally delivers 10 gtt/ml, 15 gtt/ml, or 20 gtt/ml. A microdrip set always delivers 60 gtt/ml. To calculate an infusion rate, you must first know the calibration of the drip rate for each manufacturer's product.

ADD-A-LINE SETS
Add-a-line sets can deliver intermittent secondary infusions through one or more additional Y-sites. A backcheck valve prevents backflow of the secondary solution into the primary solution. After the secondary solution has been infused, the set automatically resumes infusing the primary one.

VOLUME-CONTROL SETS
Volume-control sets — used primarily for children — deliver small, precise amounts of fluids and drugs from a volume-control chamber that's calibrated in milliliters. This chamber is placed at the top of the I.V. tubing, just above the drip chamber. Also called *burette sets*, volume-control sets are available with or without an in-line filter. They may be attached directly to the venipuncture device or connected to the Y-site of a primary I.V. administration set. Macrodrip and microdrip systems are available.

In-line filters
In-line filters are located in a segment of the I.V. tubing through which the fluid passes. In-line filters remove pathogens and parti-

(Text continues on page 42.)

40 ■ *Peripheral I.V. therapy*

Comparing I.V. administration sets

I.V. administration sets come in three major types: basic (also called *primary*), add-a-line (also called *secondary*), and volume-control. The basic set is used to administer most I.V. solutions. An add-a-line set delivers an intermittent secondary infusion through one or more additional Y-sites, or Y-ports. A volume-control set delivers small, precise amounts of solution. All three types come with vented or nonvented drip chambers.

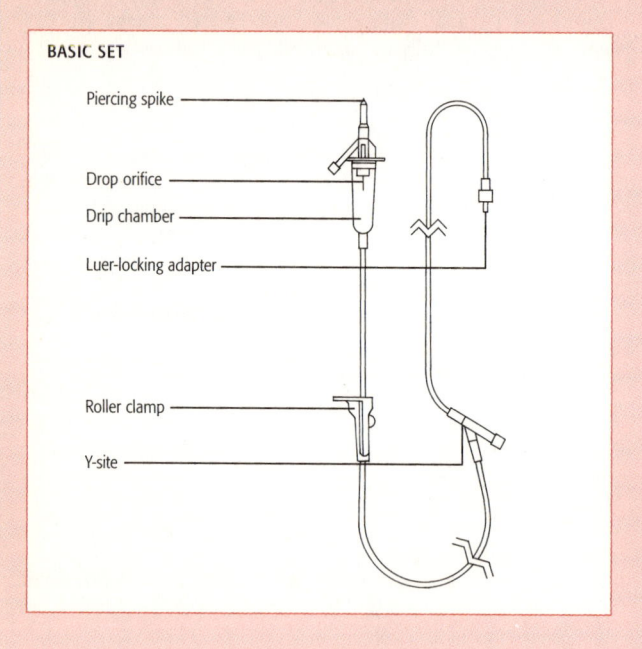

BASIC SET

- Piercing spike
- Drop orifice
- Drip chamber
- Luer-locking adapter
- Roller clamp
- Y-site

Preparing for venipuncture and infusion ■ 41

ADD-A-LINE SET

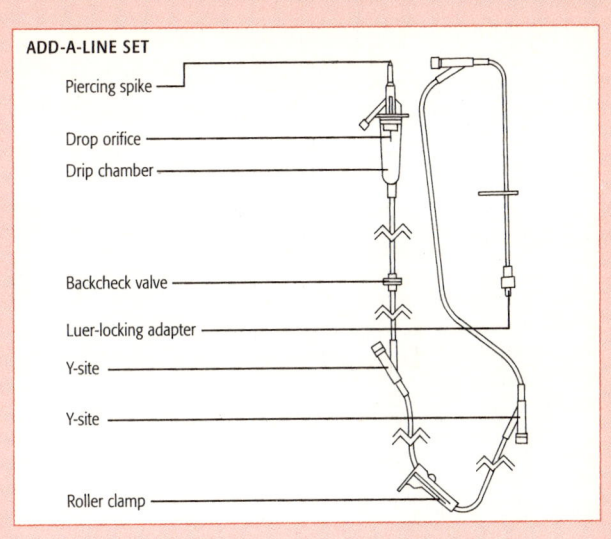

- Piercing spike
- Drop orifice
- Drip chamber
- Backcheck valve
- Luer-locking adapter
- Y-site
- Y-site
- Roller clamp

VOLUME-CONTROL SET

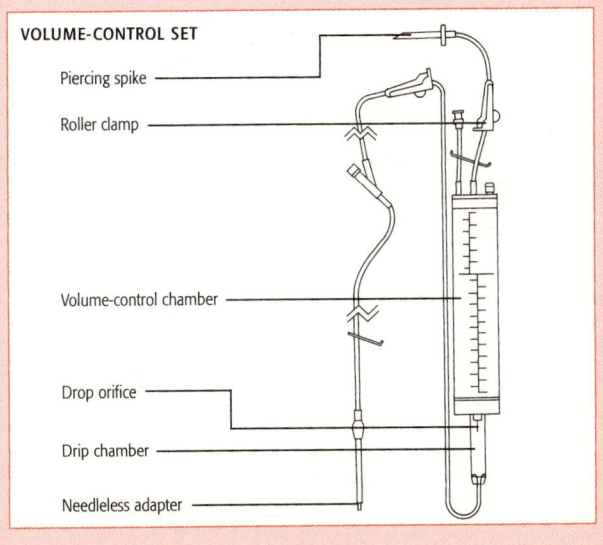

- Piercing spike
- Roller clamp
- Volume-control chamber
- Drop orifice
- Drip chamber
- Needleless adapter

cles, thus reducing the risk of infection and phlebitis. Filters also help prevent air from entering the patient's vein by venting it through the filter housing. Filters range in size from 0.2 micron (the most common) to 170 microns. Some are built into the line; others need to be added.

Most facilities have guidelines for using in-line filters; they usually include the following instructions:

- When using a filter with an infusion pump, make sure that it can withstand the pump's infusion pressure. Some filters are made for use only with gravity flow and may crack if the pressure exceeds a certain level.
- The filter should be closer to the patient than the bag.
- Carefully prime the in-line filter to eliminate all air, following the manufacturer's directions.
- Change the filter according to the manufacturer's recommendation. This helps to prevent bacteria from accumulating and releasing endotoxins and pyrogens small enough to pass through the filter into the bloodstream.

Routine use of filters increases costs; filters aren't indicated in all situations. Use an in-line filter usually when:

- treating an immunosuppressed patient
- administering total parenteral nutrition
- using additives composed of many separate particles (such as antibiotics that require reconstitution) or when administering several additives
- the risk of phlebitis is high.

Don't use a 0.2-micron filter if you're administering less than 5 mcg/ml of a low-volume drug because the filter membrane may absorb them.

PREPARING THE EQUIPMENT

After you select and gather the infusion equipment, prepare it for use. This involves inspecting the I.V. container and solution, preparing the solution, attaching and priming the administration set, and setting up the controller or infusion pump.

Inspecting the container and solution

Check that the container size and the type of I.V. solution are correct. Note the expiration date; discard an outdated solution.

Make sure that the solution container is intact. Examine a glass container for cracks or chips and a plastic container for tears or leaks. (Plastic bags usually come with an outer wrapper, which you must remove before inspecting the container.) Discard a damaged container, even if the solution appears clear. If the solution isn't clear, discard the container and notify the pharmacy or dispensing department. Solutions may vary in color, but they should never appear cloudy, turbid, or separated.

Preparing the solution

Make sure the container is labeled with the following information: your name; the patient's name, identification number, and room number; the date and time the container was hung; any additives; and the container number.

LIFE STAGES *For children, label the volume-control set instead of the container.*

After the container is labeled, use sterile technique to remove the cap or the pull tab. Don't contaminate the port.

Attaching the administration set

Make sure the administration set is correct for the patient, and for the type of I.V. container and solution you're using. Also, make sure the set has no cracks, holes, or missing clamps. If the solution container is glass, check whether it's vented or nonvented. This will determine how you prepare it before attaching it to the administration set. (Plastic containers are prepared differently.)

NONVENTED BOTTLE

When attaching a nonvented bottle to an administration set, take the following steps:

- Remove the metal cap and inner disk, if needed.
- Place the bottle on a stable surface, and wipe the rubber stopper with an alcohol swab.
- Close the flow clamp on the administration set.
- Remove the protective cap from the spike.
- Push the spike through the center of the rubber stopper. Avoid twisting or angling the spike to prevent pieces of the stopper from breaking off and falling into the solution. If the vacuum is intact you should hear a swoosh, indicating that the solution hasn't been contaminated. (You may not hear this sound if a drug has been added to the bottle.)
- Invert the bottle. If the vacuum isn't intact, discard the bottle. If it is intact, hang the bottle on the I.V. pole, about 36″ (91 cm) above the venipuncture site.

VENTED BOTTLE

When attaching a vented bottle to an administration set, take the following steps:

- Remove the metal cap and latex diaphragm to release the vacuum. If the vacuum isn't intact, discard the bottle (unless a drug has been added).
- Place the bottle on a stable surface, and wipe the rubber stopper with an alcohol swab.
- Close the flow clamp on the administration set.
- Remove the protective cap from the spike.
- Push the spike through the insertion port, which is located next to the air vent.
- Hang the bottle on the I.V. pole about 36" (91 cm) above the venipuncture site.

PLASTIC BAG
When attaching a plastic bag to an administration set, take the following steps:
- Place the bag on a flat, stable surface or hang it on an I.V. pole.
- Remove the protective cap or tear the tab from the tubing insertion port.
- Slide the flow clamp up close to the drip chamber, and close the clamp.
- Remove the protective cap from the spike.
- Hold the port carefully and firmly with one hand, and quickly insert the spike with your other hand.
- Hang the bag about 36" above the venipuncture site.

Priming the administration set
Before you prime any administration set, label it with the date and time you opened it. Make sure that you have also labeled the container. When priming a set with an electronic infusion device, the procedure is similar to priming other infusion sets. (See *Electronic infusion devices*.)

PRIMING A BASIC SET
When priming a basic set, take the following steps:
- Close the roller clamp.
- Squeeze the drip chamber until it's half full.
- Aim the end of the tubing at a receptacle to catch any solution that may overflow once the clamp is opened.
- Open the roller clamp, and allow the solution to flow through the tubing to remove the air. (Most tube coverings allow the solution to flow without having to remove the protective end.)
- Close the clamp after the solution has run through the line and all the air has been purged from the system.

Electronic infusion devices

Electronic infusion devices, such as pumps and controllers, help regulate the rate and volume of infusions, improving the safety and accuracy of drug and fluid administration.

PRIMING THE SET
Follow the steps below to prime an infusion set with an electronic infusion device:
1. Fill the drip chamber to the halfway mark.
2. Slowly open the roller clamp.
3. As gravity assists the flow, invert the chambered sections of the tubing to expel the air and fill them with the I.V. fluid or infusing solution. The chambered sections fit into the pump of the electronic infusion device; they must be filled exactly so they won't activate the air-in-line alarm during use.
4. Reinvert the pump chamber, continuing to purge the air along the fluid path and out of the tubing.

PRIMING AN ADD-A-LINE SET
Follow the same steps you would use to prime a basic set, along with these additional steps:
- As the solution flows through the tubing, invert the backcheck valves so the solution can flow into them. Tap the backcheck valve to release any trapped air bubbles.
- Straighten the tubing and continue purging air in the usual manner.

PRIMING A VOLUME-CONTROL SET
To prime a volume-control set, take the following steps:
- Attach the set to the solution container, and close the lower clamp on the I.V. tubing.
- Open the clamp between the solution container and the fluid chamber and allow about 50 ml of the solution to flow into the chamber.
- Close the upper clamp.
- Open the lower clamp and allow the solution in the chamber to flow through the remainder of the tubing. Make sure some fluid remains in the chamber so air won't fill the tubing below it.
- Close the lower clamp.
- Fill the chamber with the desired amount of solution.

USING A FILTER
If you're using a filter on any of these sets and it isn't a main part of the infusion path, attach it to the primed end of the I.V. tubing and follow the manufacturer's instructions for filling and priming it. Most filters are positioned so the solution will wet the filter membrane completely and the line will be purged of all air bubbles.

Setting up and monitoring an infusion pump
Infusion pumps help maintain a steady flow of liquid at a set rate over a specified period of time. After gathering your equipment, follow these steps:
- Attach the controller to the I.V. pole. Insert the administration spike into the I.V. container.
- Fill the drip chamber completely to prevent air bubbles from entering the tubing. To avoid fluid overload, clamp the tubing whenever the pump door is open.
- Follow the manufacturer's instructions for priming and placing the I.V. tubing.
- Be sure to flush all the air out of the tubing before connecting it to the patient; this lowers the risk of an air embolism.
- Place the infusion pump on the same side of the bed as the I.V. setup and the intended venipuncture site.
- Set the controls to the desired infusion rate or volume.
- Check the patency of the I.V. device, watch for infiltration, and monitor the accuracy of the infusion rate.

Explain the alarm system to the patient, so he isn't frightened when a change in the infusion rate triggers the alarm. Also, if infiltration occurs, disengage the device; otherwise, the pump will continue to infuse the drug into the infiltrated area.

Frequently check the infusion pump to make sure it's working properly—specifically, note the infusion rate. Monitor the patient for signs of infiltration and other complications, such as infection and air embolism.

After the equipment is up and running, you'll also need to change the tubing according to the manufacturer's instructions and your facility's policy, usually every 24 hours.

SELECTING THE INSERTION SITE
Here are some general suggestions for selecting the vein:
- Keep in mind that the most prominent veins aren't necessarily the best veins—they're typically sclerotic from previous use.

RED FLAG *Never select a vein in an edematous or impaired arm, in the arm closest to an area that's*

Preparing for venipuncture and infusion ■ 47

surgically compromised — for example, veins compromised by a mastectomy or placement of dialysis access, or in the affected arm of a patient who has had a stroke.

- Select a vein in the nondominant arm or hand.
- For subsequent venipunctures, select sites above the previously used or injured vein.
- Make sure that you rotate access sites.

RED FLAG *Don't place a catheter over the wrist; this can cause mechanical phlebitis, and the device can become dislodged.*

Commonly used veins

The veins commonly used for placement of venipuncture devices include the metacarpal, cephalic, and basilic veins, along with the branches or accessory branches that merge with them. (See *Comparing peripheral venipuncture sites,* pages 48 and 49.)

HAND AND FOREARM

Generally, the superficial veins on the back of the hand and forearm offer the most choices. The back of the hand is well supplied with small, superficial veins that can be dilated easily and usually accommodate either a needle or a catheter. The back of the forearm has long, straight veins with fairly large diameters, making them convenient sites for introducing the large-bore needles and long I.V. catheters used in prolonged I.V. therapy.

RED FLAG *If possible, avoid the antecubital fossa as the catheter may interfere with arm bending and blood sampling.*

UPPER ARMS

Veins of the hand and forearm are suitable for most drugs and solutions. For irritating drugs and solutions with a high osmolarity, the cephalic and basilic veins in the upper arm are more suitable. Be sure to check your state board of nursing practice guidelines for I.V. therapy, as many states only allow LPNs to initiate I.V. therapy in the antecubital area and below.

ARTERIES VS. VEINS

Before choosing an I.V. site, make sure it's actually a vein — not an artery. Because arteries are located deeper than veins, they're rarely damaged during venipuncture. Arteries contain bright red blood

(Text continues on page 50.)

Comparing peripheral venipuncture sites

Venipuncture sites located in the hand, forearm, foot, and leg offer various advantages and disadvantages. This chart includes some of the major benefits and drawbacks of common venipuncture sites. Check your state nurse practice act because you may be limited in which venipuncture sites you can use.

Site and location	Advantages	Disadvantages
Digital veins		
Along lateral and dorsal portions of fingers	• May be used for short-term therapy • May be used when other means aren't available	• Requires splinting fingers with a tongue blade, which decreases ability to use hand • Uncomfortable for patient • Significant risk of infiltration • Can't be used if veins in back of hand have already been used • Won't accommodate large volumes or fast I.V. rates
Metacarpal veins		
On back of hand; formed by union of digital veins between knuckles	• Easily accessible • Lie flat on back of hand; more difficult to dislodge • In adult or large child, bones of hand act as splint	• Wrist movement limited unless short catheter is used • Painful insertion likely because of large number of nerve endings in hands • Phlebitis likely at site
Accessory cephalic vein		
Along radial bone as a continuation of metacarpal veins of thumb	• Large vein excellent for venipuncture • Readily accepts large-gauge needles • Doesn't impair mobility • Doesn't require an arm board in an older child or adult	• May be difficult to position catheter flush with skin • Discomfort during movement from location of device at bend of wrist

Comparing peripheral venipuncture sites
(continued)

Site and location	Advantages	Disadvantages
CEPHALIC VEIN		
Along radial side of forearm and upper arm	• Large vein excellent for venipuncture • Readily accepts large-gauge needles • Doesn't impair mobility	• Decreased joint movement from having device close to elbow • May be difficult to stabilize the vein
MEDIAN ANTEBRACHIAL VEIN		
Rising from palm and along ulnar side of forearm	• Holds winged needles well • A last resort when no other means are available	• Painful insertion or infiltration damage possible from large number of nerve endings in area • High risk of infiltration in this area
BASILIC VEIN		
Along ulnar side of forearm and upper arm	• Accepts large-gauge needle easily • Straight, strong vein suitable for venipuncture	• Inconvenient position for patient during insertion • Painful insertion from penetration of dermal layer of skin where nerve endings are located • May be difficult to stabilize vein
ANTECUBITAL VEINS		
In antecubital fossa (median cephalic, on radial side; median basilic, on ulnar side; median cubital, which rises in front of elbow joint)	• Large vein; facilitates drawing blood • Commonly visible or palpable in children when other veins won't dilate • May be used in an emergency or as a last resort	• Difficult to splint elbow area with arm board • Veins may be small and scarred if blood has been drawn frequently from this site • Impairs patient movement and mobility

Reviewing skin and vein anatomy

Understanding the anatomy of skin and veins can help you locate appropriate venipuncture sites and perform venipunctures with minimal patient discomfort.

LAYERS OF THE SKIN

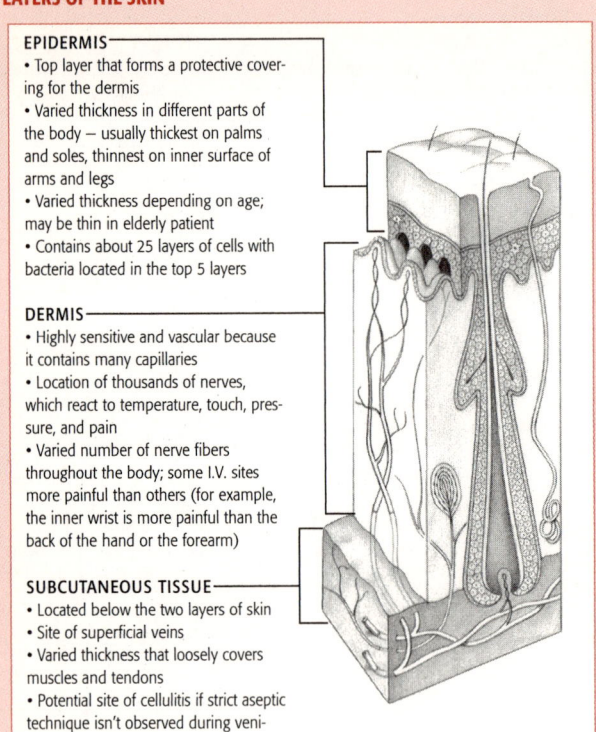

EPIDERMIS
- Top layer that forms a protective covering for the dermis
- Varied thickness in different parts of the body — usually thickest on palms and soles, thinnest on inner surface of arms and legs
- Varied thickness depending on age; may be thin in elderly patient
- Contains about 25 layers of cells with bacteria located in the top 5 layers

DERMIS
- Highly sensitive and vascular because it contains many capillaries
- Location of thousands of nerves, which react to temperature, touch, pressure, and pain
- Varied number of nerve fibers throughout the body; some I.V. sites more painful than others (for example, the inner wrist is more painful than the back of the hand or the forearm)

SUBCUTANEOUS TISSUE
- Located below the two layers of skin
- Site of superficial veins
- Varied thickness that loosely covers muscles and tendons
- Potential site of cellulitis if strict aseptic technique isn't observed during venipuncture and care of I.V. site

that flows away from the heart; veins contain dark red blood that flows toward the heart.

A single artery supplies a large area; many veins supply and remove blood from the same area. If you puncture an artery, the blood

LAYERS OF VEINS

TUNICA INTIMA (INNER LAYER)
- Inner elastic endothelial lining made up of layers of smooth, flat cells, which allow blood cells and platelets to flow smoothly through the blood vessels (unnecessary movement of the venous access device may scratch or roughen this inner surface, causing thrombus formation)
- Valves in this layer located in the semilunar folds of the endothelium (valves prevent backflow and ensure that blood flows toward the heart)

TUNICA MEDIA (MIDDLE LAYER)
- Muscular and elastic tissue
- Location of vasoconstrictor and vasodilator nerve fibers that stimulate the veins to contract and relax (these fibers are responsible for venous spasm that can occur as the result of anxiety or infusion of I.V. fluids that are too cold)

TUNICA ADVENTITIA (OUTER LAYER)
- Connective tissue that surrounds and supports the vessel and holds it together
- Reduced thickness and amount of connective tissue with age, resulting in fragile veins

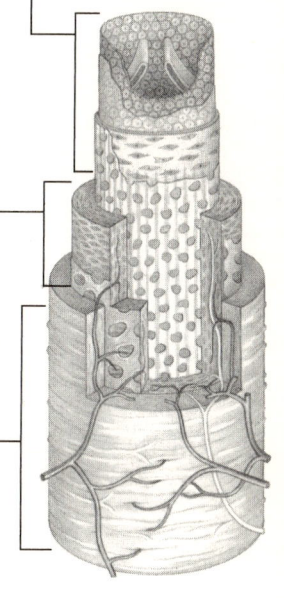

pulsates from the site; if you puncture a vein, the blood flows slowly. (See *Reviewing skin and vein anatomy*.)

VALVES
All major veins have valves, but they're usually apparent only in long, straight arm veins or in large, well-developed veins that have good tone. If possible, don't let the tip of the venipuncture device terminate near a valve — it might affect the flow rate.

Selection guidelines
When selecting an I.V. site, choose distal veins first, unless the solution is very irritating (for example, 40 mEq or more of potassium chloride). Generally, your best choice is a peripheral vein that's full and pliable and appears long enough to accommodate the length of the intended catheter. It should be large enough to allow blood flow around the catheter; this will minimize venous lumen irritation. If the patient has an area that's bruised, tender, or phlebitic, choose a vein nearby. Avoid bending areas.

VEINS TO AVOID
Veins in the following places are best to avoid:
- the legs (circulation may be easily compromised and increase the risk for phlebitis)
- the inner wrist and arm (they're small and uncomfortable for the patient)
- the affected arm of a mastectomy patient
- an arm with an arteriovenous shunt or fistula
- an arm being treated for thrombosis or cellulitis.

VEIN SIZE AND HEALTH
The size and health (tone) of the vein help determine how long the venipuncture device can remain in place before irritation develops. However, the key to determining how long the venous access device will remain functional is the effect of the fluid or drug on the vein. Drugs and solutions with high osmolarity and high or low pH will cause vein irritation sooner. Concentrated solutions of drugs and rapid infusion rates can also affect how long the I.V. site remains free of pain or irritation.

SELECTING THE INFUSION DEVICE
Basically, you should select the device with the shortest length and the smallest diameter that allows for proper administration of the therapy. Other considerations include:
- length of time the device will stay in place
- type of therapy
- type of procedure or surgery to be performed

- patient's age and activity level
- type of solution used (blood, for instance, will require a larger-gauge device)
- available veins.

Infusion devices

The two most commonly used devices are plastic catheter sets and winged steel needle infusion sets. As a rule, plastic catheters allow the patient to move more and are less prone to infiltration than steel needles. However, they're more difficult to insert. (See *Comparing basic venipuncture devices,* pages 54 and 55.)

OVER-THE-NEEDLE CATHETER

An over-the-needle catheter, also known as a *needleless system,* is the most commonly used device for peripheral I.V. therapy. It consists of a plastic outer tube and an inner needle that extends just beyond the catheter. It's available in lengths of 1" and 1¼", with gauges ranging from 14 to 26. Longer-length models, used mainly in the operating room, are for insertion into a deep vein. (See *Guide to needle and catheter gauges,* page 56.)

The needle is removed after insertion, leaving the catheter in place. Typically, you should change over-the-needle catheters every 2 or 3 days, depending on the facility's policy and procedures. If the patient has poor venous access and therapy is to be continued indefinitely, consult the physician about line-placement alternatives.

WINGED-INFUSION SETS

Winged-infusion sets come in two basic types: an over-the-needle catheter and a steel needle. Both have flexible wings you can grasp when inserting the device. Once the device is in place, the wings lie flat and can be taped to the surrounding skin.

Winged over-the-needle catheters have short, small-bore tubing between the catheter and the hub. The catheter stays in place after the needle is removed. This type of catheter is available in a ¾" length for wider gauges and is especially useful for hard veins and for intermittent or one-time drug administration when I.V. access isn't otherwise needed.

Commonly called *butterfly needles,* winged steel needle catheters have no hub and lie flat on the skin, which makes taping easy. These devices range in size from 19G to 27G and are about ¾" long. Originally designed for use in children or elderly patients, the winged steel needle should be used when a patient is in stable condition, has adequate veins, and requires I.V. fluids or drugs for only

(Text continues on page 57.)

Comparing basic venipuncture devices

OVER-THE-NEEDLE CATHETER
PURPOSE
- Long-term therapy for the active or agitated patient

ADVANTAGES
- Inadvertent puncture of vein less likely than with a winged steel-needle set
- More comfortable for the patient
- Radiopaque thread for easy location
- Syringe attached to some units that permits easy check of blood return and prevents air from entering the vessel on insertion
- Safety needles that prevent accidental needle sticks
- Activity-restricting device, such as arm board, rarely required

DISADVANTAGES
- Difficult to insert
- Extra care required to ensure that needle and catheter are inserted into vein

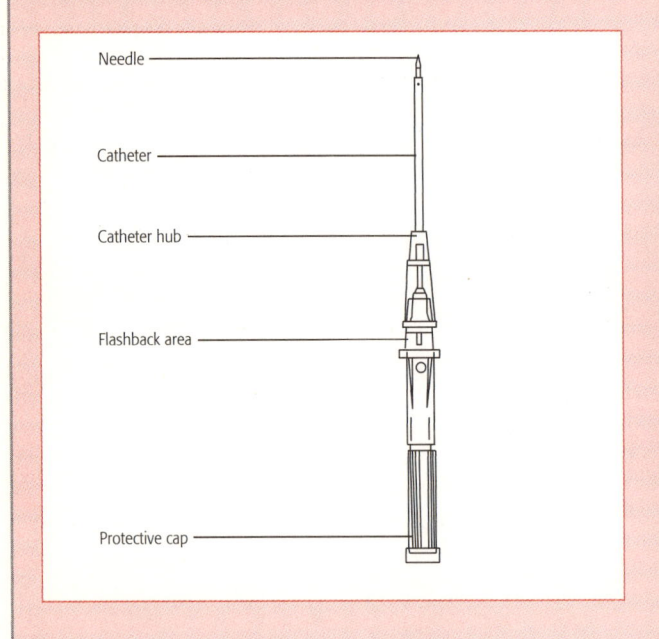

Needle

Catheter

Catheter hub

Flashback area

Protective cap

WINGED STEEL NEEDLE SET
PURPOSE
- Short-term therapy (such as a single-dose infusion) for cooperative adult patient
- Therapy of any duration for an infant or child or for an elderly patient with fragile or sclerotic veins

ADVANTAGES
- Easiest intravascular device to insert because needle is thin-walled and extremely sharp
- Ideal for nonirritating I.V. push drugs
- Available with catheter that can be left in place like over-the-needle catheter

DISADVANTAGE
- Infiltration easily caused if rigid needle-winged infusion device is used

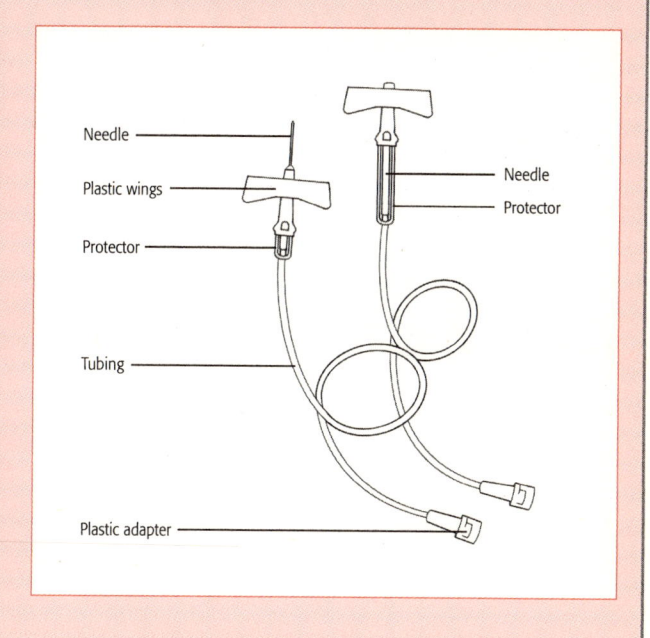

- Needle
- Plastic wings
- Protector
- Tubing
- Plastic adapter
- Needle
- Protector

Guide to needle and catheter gauges

How do you know which gauge needle and catheter to use for your patient? The answer depends on the patient's age, his condition, and the type of infusion he's receiving. This table lists the uses and nursing considerations for various gauges.

GAUGE	USES	NURSING CONSIDERATIONS
16	• Adolescents and adults • Major surgery • Trauma • Whenever large amounts of fluids must be infused rapidly	• Painful insertion • Requires large vein
18	• Older children, adolescents, and adults • Administration of blood and blood components and other viscous infusions • Routinely used preoperatively • To deliver hydration	• Painful insertion • Requires large vein
20	• Children, adolescents, and adults • Suitable for most I.V. infusions, blood, blood components, and other viscous infusions	• Commonly used
22	• Toddlers, children, adolescents, and adults (especially elderly) • Suitable for most I.V. infusions • Total parental nutrition and lipid infusions • To deliver hydration	• Easier to insert into small veins • Commonly used for most infusions
24, 26	• Neonates, infants, toddlers, school-age children, adolescents, and adults (especially elderly) • Suitable for most infusions, but flow rates are slower • Commonly used for chemotherapy infusions	• For extremely small veins — for example, small veins of fingers or veins of inner arms in elderly patients • May be difficult to insert into tough skin

Venipuncture variations

Here are some common variations on venipuncture devices.

WINGED INFUSION SETS WITH CATHETER
Winged infusion sets sometimes have an over-the-needle catheter plus short, small-bore tubing between the catheter and hub. These catheters are available in a ¾" length for smaller gauges and a 1" length for larger ones. They're especially useful for hand veins or areas that require angled insertions.

WINGED AND Y-SHAPED
Another type of winged infusion set has a Y-shaped design with a latex cap and is available in 16G to 24G. Because it has two ports, this set can be used for intermittent infusion while a continuous I.V. solution is infusing, or for simultaneous infusion of two compatible solutions. Recent design changes have reduced the amount of latex in the Y-site, a consideration for staff or patients with latex allergies.

DUAL-LUMEN CATHETER
For simultaneous infusion of two *incompatible* solutions, you might use the dual-lumen catheter. This set consists of side-by-side catheters that come together at a single tip. It's also useful for infusing more than one drug over a short period and for drawing blood. Recommended only for arm veins, the dual-lumen catheter requires greater insertion skills than other venous access devices.

---

a short time. They're also ideal for single I.V. push injections. (For a description of this and other variations on I.V. devices, see *Venipuncture variations*.)

INTERMITTENT DEVICE
Any infusion device that includes a catheter can be made into an intermittent infusion device by placing an access cap over the catheter's adapter end. These caps are commonly called "locks" and a saline solution is flushed into them to keep the device patent. Typically, the cap is a luer-locking attachment or add-on. Intermittent infusion devices should be flushed with saline solution before and after each use, at least once per day, or according to the facility's policy and procedures.

Performing venipuncture

To perform a venipuncture, you need to dilate the vein, prepare the access site, and insert the device. After the infusion starts, you can complete the I.V. placement by securing the device with tape or a transparent semipermeable dressing.

DILATING THE VEIN

To dilate or distend a vein effectively, you need to use a tourniquet, which traps blood in the veins by applying enough pressure to impede venous flow. A properly distended vein should appear and feel round, firm, and fully filled with blood as well as rebound when gently compressed. Because the amount of trapped blood depends on circulation, a patient who is hypotensive, very cold, or experiencing vasomotor changes (such as septic shock) may have inadequate filling of the peripheral blood vessels.

Before applying the tourniquet, place the patient's arm in a position lower than his heart to increase capillary flow to the lower arm and hand. If his skin is cold, warm it by rubbing and stroking his arm or by covering the entire arm with warm moist towels for 5 to 10 minutes. As soon as you remove the warm towels, apply the tourniquet and continue to perform the insertion procedure.

Applying a tourniquet

The ideal tourniquet is one that can be secured easily, doesn't roll into a thin band, stays relatively flat, and releases easily. The most common type is a soft rubber band about 2″ (5 cm) wide. Other types use Velcro or a catch mechanism to anchor them. (See *Applying a tourniquet*.)

Once you have applied the tourniquet about 6″ to 8″ (15 to 20 cm) above the intended site, have the patient open and close his fist tightly four to six times to distend the vein. If necessary, gently flick the skin over the vein with one or two short taps of your forefinger. This is less traumatic than slapping the skin, but it achieves the same result. If the vein still feels small and uniform, release the tourniquet, reapply it, and reassess the intended access site. If the vein still isn't adequately distended, remove the tourniquet; apply a warm, moist towel for 5 minutes; then reapply the tourniquet. This is especially helpful if the patient's skin feels cool.

RED FLAG *A tourniquet that's kept in place too long or is applied too tightly may cause increased bruising, especially in elderly patients whose veins are fragile. Release the*

Applying a tourniquet

To safely apply a tourniquet, follow these steps:

1. Place the tourniquet under the patient's arm, about 6" (15 cm) above the venipuncture site. Position the arm on the middle of the tourniquet.
2. Bring the ends of the tourniquet together, placing one on top of the other.
3. Holding one end on top of the other, lift and stretch the tourniquet and tuck the top tail under the bottom tail. Don't allow the tourniquet to loosen.
4. Tie the tourniquet smoothly and snugly; be careful not to pinch the patient's skin or pull his arm hair.

NO MORE THAN 2 MINUTES
Leave the tourniquet in place for no more than 2 minutes. If you can't find a suitable vein and prepare the venipuncture site in this amount of time, release the tourniquet for a few minutes. Then reapply it and continue the procedure. You may need to apply the tourniquet, find the vein, remove the tourniquet, prepare the site, and then reapply the tourniquet for the venipuncture.

AS FLAT AS POSSIBLE
Keep the tourniquet as flat as possible. It should be snug but not uncomfortably tight. If it's too tight, it will impede arterial as well as venous blood flow. Check the patient's radial pulse. If you can't feel it, the tourniquet is too tight and must be loosened. Also loosen and reapply the tourniquet if the patient complains of severe tightness.

---

tourniquet as soon as you have placed the venipuncture device in the vein.

Ideally, your facility's infection-control guidelines will call for tourniquets to be discarded after one use. When available, use latex-free tourniquets to reduce the chance of allergic reaction.

PREPARING THE ACCESS SITE

Before performing venipuncture, you need to clean the site and stabilize the vein; you may also need to administer a local anesthetic.

Cleaning the venipuncture site

Wash your hands; then put on gloves. If necessary, snip the hair over the insertion site to make the veins and the site easier to see and reduce pain when the tape is removed. Avoid shaving the patient. Microabrasion of the skin may occur, increasing the risk of infection.

Clean the skin with 2% chlorhexidine or a thin coat of 10% povidone-iodine solution. (Other antimicrobial solutions are tincture of iodine 2% and 70% alcohol.) Using a swab, start at the center of the insertion site and move outward with a side-to-side motion. Be careful not to go over an area you have already cleaned. Allow the solution 30 to 60 seconds to dry thoroughly.

Using a local anesthetic

If an anesthetic is ordered and your state practice guidelines allow you to administer a local anesthetic, first check with the patient and review his record for an allergy to lidocaine, iodine, or any other drugs. Then describe the procedure to him and explain that it will reduce the discomfort of the venipuncture.

Next, administer the local anesthetic. You'll administer only a small amount, and the anesthetic will begin to work in 2 or 3 seconds. Lidocaine anesthetizes the site to pain but allows the patient to feel touch and pressure. Normal saline solution has also proven effective. (See *Administering a local anesthetic*.)

LIFE STAGES A transdermal analgesic cream is a good choice for anesthetizing I.V. sites in children. Like injectable anesthetics, transdermal analgesic cream reduces pain, but the patient still feels pressure and touch. To be effective, a transdermal analgesic cream should be applied 60 minutes before insertion of the venous access device.

Stabilizing the vein

Stabilizing the vein helps ensure a successful venipuncture the first time and decreases the chances of bruising. If the tip of the venipuncture device repeatedly probes a moving vein wall, it can nick the vein and cause it to leak blood. When this happens, the vein can't be reused immediately and a new venipuncture site must be found, exposing the patient to the risk and discomfort of another needle puncture.

To stabilize the vein, stretch the skin and hold it taut, then lightly press it with your fingertips about 1½" (4 cm) from the insertion site.

RED FLAG Never touch the prepared site or you'll recontaminate it.

The vein should feel round, firm, fully engorged, and resilient. Remove your fingertips. If the vein returns to its original position and appears larger than it did before you applied the tourniquet, it's adequately distended.

Performing venipuncture ■ 61

Administering a local anesthetic

A local anesthetic may be used when starting peripheral I.V. therapy. If a local anesthetic is ordered, follow the steps below.
- Using a U-100 insulin syringe with a 27G needle, draw 0.1 ml of lidocaine 1% without epinephrine.
- Clean the venipuncture site.
- Insert the needle next to the vein, introducing about one-third of it into the skin at a 30-degree angle. The side approach carries less risk of accidental vein puncture (indicated by blood appearing in the syringe). But if the vein is deep, inject the lidocaine over the top of it. To make sure that you don't inject lidocaine into the vein — thus allowing it to circulate systemically — aspirate to check for a blood return. If this occurs, withdraw the needle and begin the procedure again.
- Hold your thumb on the plunger of the syringe during insertion to avoid unnecessary movement when the needle is under the skin.
- Without aspirating, quickly inject the lidocaine until a small wheal appears (as shown). You may not have to administer the entire amount in the syringe.
- Quickly withdraw the syringe and massage the wheal with an alcohol swab. This will make the wheal disappear so the vein won't be hidden — although you'll see a small pinprick of blood. The skin numbness will last about 30 minutes.
- Insert the venous access device into the vein.

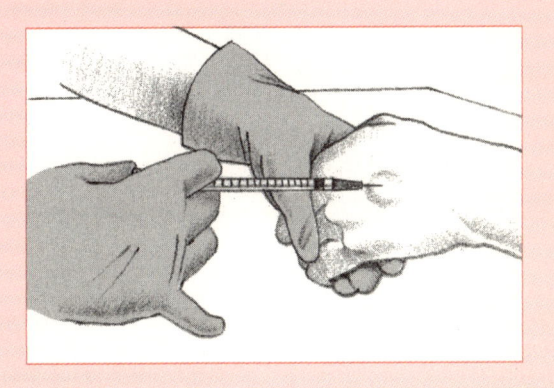

To help prevent the vein from moving, apply adequate traction with your nondominant hand to hold the skin and vein in place. This is particularly helpful in elderly patients with loose skin and loosely anchored veins. (See *How to stabilize veins*, page 62.)

How to stabilize veins

To help ensure successful venipuncture, you need to stabilize the patient's vein by stretching the skin and holding it taut. The stretching technique you'll use varies with the venipuncture site. This chart lists the various venipuncture sites along with a description of the stretching technique used for each.

VEIN	STRETCHING TECHNIQUE
Metacarpal (hand) veins	Stretch the patient's hand and wrist downward, and hold the skin taut with your thumb.
Cephalic vein above wrist	Stretch the patient's fist laterally downward, and immobilize the skin with the thumb of your other hand.
Basilic vein at outer arm	Have the patient flex his elbow. While standing behind the flexed arm, retract the skin away from the site, and anchor the vein with your thumb. As an alternative, rotate the patient's extended lower arm inward, and approach the vein from behind the arm. (This position may be difficult for the patient to maintain.)
Inner aspect of wrist	Extend the patient's open hand backward from the wrist. Anchor the vein with your thumb below the insertion site.
Inner arm	Anchor the vein with your thumb above the wrist.
Antecubital fossa	Have the patient extend his arm completely. Anchor the skin with your thumb, about 2" to 3" (5 to 7.5 cm) below the antecubital fossa.

INSERTING THE DEVICE

When you have prepared the venipuncture site, you're ready to insert the infusion device. The process involves three steps: positioning, inserting, and advancing. You might also need to add an intermittent infusion device, to use deep veins rather than superficial, or to collect a blood sample.

Positioning the infusion device

While still wearing gloves, use the appropriate method for the type of infusion device being used.

OVER-THE-NEEDLE CATHETER
- Grasp the plastic hub with your dominant hand, remove the cover, and examine the device. If the edge isn't smooth, discard the device and obtain another.
- Insert the device, bevel up, through the skin and into the vein; then lower the hub portion until it's almost parallel to the skin.
- Advance the device to at least half its length, at which point you should see blood in the flashback chamber.
- Remove the needle (stylette).
- Apply the cap or attach the I.V. tubing, and then advance the catheter to its hub.

WINGED INFUSION DEVICE
- Hold the edges of the wings with your thumb and forefinger, with the bevel facing upward.
- Squeeze the wings together.
- Remove the protective cover from the needle, being careful not to contaminate the steel needle or the catheter.

Inserting the infusion device
Tell the patient that you're about to insert the device. Ask him to remain still and to refrain from pulling away. Explain that the initial needle stick will hurt but will quickly subside.
- Then insert the device, using the direct approach. Place the bevel up and enter the skin directly over the vein at a 5- to 15-degree angle (deeper veins require a wider angle).
- When you insert the device, use a steady, smooth motion while keeping the skin taut. Usually, you'll know the device is in the vein because you'll meet resistance during insertion and see blood return in the flashback chamber. (You may not see a rapid blood return with a small vein.)
- Don't expect to always feel a "pop" or a sense of release when the device enters the vein. This usually occurs only when a larger-gauge venipuncture device (20G or more) enters a large, thick-walled vein or when the patient has good tissue tone.
- As soon as the device enters the vein, lower the back end of the adapter until it's almost parallel with the skin. This lifts the tip of the needle so it doesn't penetrate the opposite wall of the vein.

Advancing the infusion device
You can advance the catheter before starting the infusion or while infusing the I.V. solution. The advantage of advancing the catheter before starting the infusion is that it commonly results in less blood

being spilled. The advantage of advancing the catheter while the I.V. is infusing is that it reduces the risk of puncturing the vein wall because the catheter is advanced without the steel needle and the rapid flow dilates the vein. However, this method increases the risk of infection. The Centers for Disease Control and Prevention recommends using needleless systems to decrease the risk.

ADVANCING THE CATHETER BEFORE STARTING THE INFUSION
- Release the tourniquet.
- While stabilizing the vein with one hand, use the other to advance the catheter up to the hub.
- Remove the inner needle.
- Apply pressure with your fingers to the catheter (to minimize blood exposure) and, using aseptic technique, attach the I.V. tubing.

ADVANCING THE CATHETER WHILE INFUSING
- Release the tourniquet and remove the inner needle (stylette).
- Using aseptic technique, attach the I.V. tubing and begin the infusion.
- While stabilizing the vein with one hand, use the other to advance the catheter into the vein.
- When the catheter is advanced, slow the I.V. flow rate.

USING A WINGED STEEL NEEDLE INFUSION SET
- Advance the needle fully, if possible, and hold it in place.
- Release the tourniquet, slightly open the administration set clamp, and check for free flow or infiltration.
- Next, tape the infusion set in place, using the wings as an anchor to prevent catheter movement, which could cause irritation and phlebitis.
- When using an over-the-needle winged infusion set, you can advance the catheter using either of the methods described above.

COMPLETING THE INSERTION
- Securely tape the device and clean the skin if necessary.
- Cover the access site with a transparent dressing or the dressing used by your facility.
- If your facility's policy and procedures require doing so, further stabilize the device.
- Dispose of the inner needle in a nonpermeable receptacle.
- Regulate the flow rate; then remove your gloves and wash your hands.

Using an intermittent infusion device

Also called a *saline lock,* an intermittent infusion device may be used when venous access must be maintained for intermittent use and a continuous infusion isn't necessary. This device keeps the access device sterile and prevents blood and other fluids from leaking from an open end. Much like the administration-set injection port, the intermittent injection cap is self-sealing after the needle or needleless injector is removed. The ends of these devices are universal in size and fit the female end of any catheter or tubing designed for infusion therapy. Caps should have a luer-locking design to prevent disconnections.

The intermittent infusion device can be filled with dilute saline solution to expel air from the equipment. This makes it possible to maintain venous access in patients who must receive I.V. drugs regularly or intermittently but don't require a continuous infusion.

BENEFITS AND DISADVANTAGES
The intermittent infusion device has many benefits.
- It minimizes the risk of fluid overload and electrolyte imbalance that may be associated with a continuous infusion.
- By eliminating the continuous use of I.V. solution containers and administration sets, it reduces the risk of contamination and lowers costs.
- It allows for patient mobility, which helps reduce anxiety.

The intermittent infusion device has one clear disadvantage. If the device isn't flushed to ensure patency before and after the drug is infused, the device may become occluded.

RED FLAG If the patient feels a burning sensation as you inject the saline solution, stop the injection and check the catheter placement. If it's in the vein, inject the solution at a slower rate to minimize irritation.

If the physician orders I.V. infusion to be stopped, you can convert the existing line from a continuous to an intermittent infusion device. Just disconnect the I.V. tubing and insert an adapter plug into the device that's already in place. (See *From continuous to intermittent,* page 66.)

Inserting the infusion device into a deep vein

If a superficial vein isn't available, insert the infusion device into a deep vein that isn't visible, using the following steps:
- Wash your hands and put on gloves.
- Palpate the area with your fingertips until you feel the vein.

> **From continuous to intermittent**
>
> The male adapter plug shown below allows you to convert an existing I.V. line into an intermittent infusion device.
>
> To make the conversion:
> 1. Prime the male adapter plug with saline solution.
> 2. Clamp the I.V. tubing and remove the administration set from the catheter or needle hub.
> 3. Insert a male adapter plug.
> 4. Flush the access with the remaining solution to prevent occlusion.
>
> The male luer-locking adapter plug twists into place.

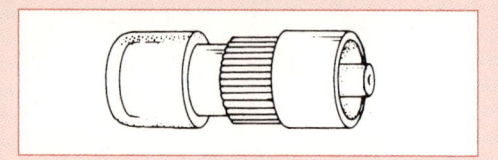

- Clean the skin over the vein with an approved cleaning solution such as chlorhexidine, swiping in a side-to-side motion.
- Aim the device directly over the intended vein, stretching the skin with your gloved fingertips, and insert the venipuncture device at a 15-degree angle to the skin.
- Insert the device one-half to two-thirds its length; that way you'll make sure that the needle and the catheter are in the vein lumen.
- When you see blood in the flashback chamber, remove the inner steel needle and advance the catheter with or without infusing fluid.

Collecting a blood sample

If a blood sample is ordered, you can collect it while performing the venipuncture. First, gather the necessary equipment: one or more evacuated tubes, a 20G needle, an appropriate-size syringe without a needle, and a protective pad. (See *Taking a blood sample.*)

SECURING THE INFUSION DEVICE

After the infusion begins, you need to secure the infusion device at the insertion site. You can do this with tape or a transparent semipermeable dressing.

Taking a blood sample

To smoothly and safely collect a blood sample, follow these steps after assembling your equipment and making the venipuncture:

- Place a pad underneath the site to protect the bed linens.
- If you're using an over-the-needle device, remove the inner needle when the infusion device is correctly placed.
- Leave the tourniquet tied.
- Attach the syringe to the infusion device's hub, and withdraw the appropriate amount of blood.
- Release the tourniquet and disconnect the syringe.
- Quickly attach the saline lock or I.V. tubing, regulate the infusion rate, and stabilize the device.
- Attach a 19G needle or needleless device to the syringe, and insert the blood into the evacuated tubes.
- Properly dispose of the needle and syringe, and then complete I.V. line placement.

Applying tape

Stabilize the device and keep the hub from moving by using a standard taping method, such as the chevron, U, and H methods. (See *Taping techniques,* page 68.)

Use as little tape as possible, and don't let the tape ends meet. This reduces the risk of a tourniquet effect if infiltration occurs. Remove any hair from around the access area. Besides improving visibility and reducing pain when the tape is removed, this helps decrease colonization by bacteria present on the hair. Don't let the tape cover the patient's skin beyond the infusion device's entry site. This could hide swelling and redness, signs of impending complications.

If the patient has had a previous sensitivity reaction to tape, use a nonallergenic tape, preferably one that's lightweight and easy to remove. Paper tape usually isn't satisfactory for I.V. sites because it shreds and is difficult to remove after prolonged contact with skin and body heat.

Applying a transparent dressing

To prevent infection, nurses in many health care facilities cover the insertion site with a transparent, semipermeable dressing. This dressing allows air to pass through but is impervious to microorganisms. (For instructions, see *How to apply a transparent semipermeable dressing,* page 69.)

Taping techniques

If you use tape to secure the venous access device to the insertion site, use one of these methods.

CHEVRON METHOD
1. Cut a long strip of ½" tape. Place it sticky side up under the hub.
2. Cross the ends of the tape over the hub, and secure the tape to the patient's skin on the opposite sides of the hub, as shown at right.
3. Apply a piece of 1" tape across the two wings of the chevron. Loop the tubing and secure it with another piece of 1" tape. Once a dressing is secured, apply a label. On the label, write the date and time of insertion, type and gauge of the needle, and your initials.

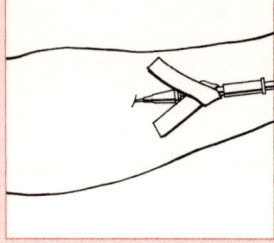

U METHOD
1. Cut a strip of ½" tape. With the sticky side up, place it under the hub of the catheter.
2. Bring each side of the tape up, folding it over the wings of the catheter, as shown at right. Press it down, parallel to the hub.
3. Next, apply tape to stabilize the catheter. After a dressing is secured, apply a label. On the label, write the date and time of insertion, type and gauge of the catheter, and your initials.

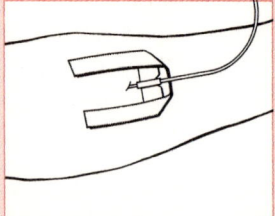

H METHOD
1. Cut three strips of ½" tape.
2. Place one strip of tape over each wing, keeping the tape parallel to the catheter.
3. Place the third strip of tape perpendicular to the first two, as shown at right. Put the tape directly on top of the wings. Make sure that the catheter is secure, and then apply a dressing and label. On the label, write the date and time of insertion, type and gauge of the catheter, and your initials.

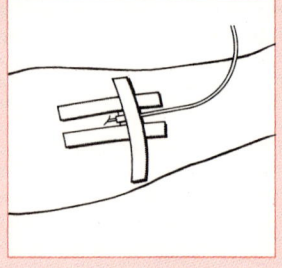

> **BEST PRACTICE**
>
> ## How to apply a transparent semipermeable dressing
>
> Here's how to apply a transparent semipermeable dressing, which allows for visual assessment of the catheter insertion site:
> - Make sure the insertion site is clean and dry.
> - Remove the dressing from the package and, using aseptic technique, remove the protective seal. Avoid touching the sterile surface.
> - Place the dressing directly over the insertion site and the hub, as shown. Don't cover the tubing. Also, don't stretch the dressing; doing so may cause itching.
> - Tuck the dressing around and under the catheter hub to make the site occlusive to microorganisms.
> - To remove the dressing, grasp one corner, and then lift and stretch.

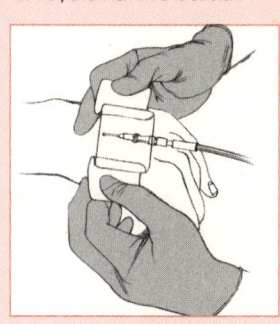

If this dressing remains intact, daily changes aren't necessary. Other advantages include fewer skin reactions and a clearly visible insertion site (especially helpful in detecting early signs of phlebitis and infiltration). The dressing is waterproof so it protects the site from contamination if it gets wet. In addition, because the dressing adheres well to the skin, there is less chance of accidentally dislodging the infusion device.

Using a stretch net
You can make the infusion device more secure by applying a stretch net to the affected limb. (If you'll be using the net on the patient's hand, cut a hole in the net sleeve for his thumb.) The net reduces the risk of accidental dislodgment, especially with patients who are confused or very active, and cuts down on the amount of tape needed to prevent dislodgment.

Using an arm board
An arm board is an immobilization device that helps secure correct infusion-device positioning and prevents unnecessary motion that could cause infiltration or inflammation. This immobilization device

is sometimes necessary when the insertion site is near a joint or in the back of the hand. It's also used with a restraint for confused or disoriented patients.

__RED FLAG__ Because it's an immobilization device, the use of an arm board may be restricted by state or facility policies, so check first. Better yet, don't place the tip of the infusion device in a bending area. Then you won't need an arm board.

To determine whether an arm board is called for, move your patient's arm through its full range of motion (ROM) while watching the I.V. infusion rate. If the flow stops during movement, you may need to use the arm board to prevent bending of the arm. Choose one that's long enough to prevent bending and extension at the tip of the device. If necessary, cover it with a soft material before you secure it to the patient's arm. Make sure that you can still observe the insertion site.

__RED FLAG__ An arm board applied too tightly can cause nerve and tendon damage. If you need to use an arm board, remove it periodically so the patient can perform ROM exercises and you can better observe for complications from restricted activity and infusion therapy.

Maintaining peripheral I.V. therapy

After starting an I.V. infusion, focus on maintaining therapy and preventing complications. This involves both routine and special-care measures, as well as discontinuing the infusion when therapy is completed. Also, you should be prepared to meet the special needs of pediatric, elderly, or home care patients who require I.V. therapy.

ROUTINE CARE

Routine care helps prevent complications. It also gives you an opportunity to observe the I.V. site for signs of inflammation or infection—two of the most common complications. Perform this care according to your facility's policy and procedures. Wash your hands and wear gloves whenever you work near the venipuncture site.

Changing the dressing

The insertion site should be inspected and palpated daily through the intact dressing for tenderness. Depending on your facility's policy, gauze dressings should be changed routinely every 48 hours. A

Changing a peripheral I.V. dressing

To change a peripheral I.V. dressing, follow these steps:
- Wash your hands and put on sterile gloves.
- Hold the needle or catheter in place with your nondominant hand to prevent movement or dislodgment that could lead to infiltration; then, gently remove the tape and the dressing.
- Assess the venipuncture site for signs of infection (redness and tenderness), infiltration (coolness, blanching, edema), and thrombophlebitis (redness, firmness, pain along the path of the vein, edema).
- If you detect any of the above signs, apply pressure to the area with a sterile gauze pad and remove the catheter or needle. Maintain pressure on the area until the bleeding stops, and then apply an adhesive bandage. Using new equipment, insert the I.V. access device at another site.
- If you don't detect complications, hold the needle or catheter at the hub and carefully clean around the site with an alcohol swab or other approved solution. Work in a swiping motion to avoid introducing pathogens into the cleaned area. Allow the area to dry completely.
- Retape the device and apply a transparent semipermeable dressing, if available, or apply gauze and secure it.

---

transparent semipermeable dressing should be changed whenever its integrity is compromised because it has become soiled, wet, or loose.

Before performing a dressing change, gather this equipment:
- povidone-iodine or alcohol swab
- adhesive bandage, sterile 2″ × 2″ gauze pad, or transparent semipermeable dressing
- 1″ clean adhesive tape
- sterile gloves.

To change a dressing, follow the steps outlined in *Changing a peripheral I.V. dressing*.

Changing the I.V. solution

To avoid microbial growth, don't allow an I.V. container to hang for more than 24 hours. Before changing the I.V. container, check the new one for cracks, leaks, and other damage. Also check the solution for discoloration, turbidity, and particulates. Note the date and time the solution was mixed and the expiration date.

After washing your hands, clamp the line, remove the spike from the old container, and quickly insert the spike into the new

Changing the administration set

To quickly change the administration set for a peripheral infusion, follow these steps:
- Wash your hands and put on gloves.
- Reduce the I.V. infusion rate. Then, remove the old spike from the container, and place the cover of the new spike over it loosely.
- Keeping the old spike upright and above the patient's heart level, insert the new spike into the I.V. container and prime the system.
- Place a sterile gauze pad under the needle or hub of the plastic catheter to create a sterile field.
- Disconnect the old tubing from the infusion device, being careful not to dislodge or move the device. If you have trouble disconnecting the old tubing, try one of these techniques: use a pair of hemostats to hold the hub securely while twisting and removing the end of the tubing, or grasp the infusion device with one pair of hemostats and the hard plastic of the luer-locking end of the administration set with another pair and pull the hemostats in opposite directions. Don't clamp the hemostats shut; this may crack the tubing adapter or the infusion device.
- Using aseptic technique, quickly attach the new primed tubing to the device.
- Adjust the flow to the prescribed rate.
- Label the new tubing with the date and time of the change.

one. Then hang the new container and adjust the flow rate as prescribed.

Changing the administration set

Change the administration set according to your facility's policy (usually every 72 hours if it's a primary infusion line) and whenever you note or suspect contamination. If possible, change the set when you start a new infusion device during routine site rotation.

Before changing the set, gather these items:
- an I.V. administration set
- a sterile 2″ × 2″ gauze pad
- adhesive tape for labeling or appropriate labeling tapes supplied by the facility
- gloves.

Then follow the guidelines set out in *Changing the administration set*.

Changing the I.V. site
As a standard of care, rotate the I.V. site every 48 to 72 hours, if possible. Limited venous access sometimes prevents you from changing sites this often. If that's the case, notify the physician of the need to deviate from normal practice and be sure to document the reasons. Obtain an order to extend the dwell time of the current access site, but remember to monitor more frequently for redness, pain, or swelling. Change the entire system, including the venipuncture device, if you detect signs of thrombophlebitis, cellulitis, or I.V. therapy-related bacteremia. Finally, document the procedure.

Adding infusions to a primary line
To piggyback an I.V. drug into a primary line, use an add-a-line administration set. To infuse two compatible solutions simultaneously, connect an administration set with an attached needleless access catheter (or one with a needle) to the secondary solution container and prime the tubing. (Using needles to apply a second infusion creates increased risks associated with needle sticks, so exercise extreme caution.) Hang the container at the same level as the primary solution.

Next, clean a Y-site in the lower part of the primary tubing, using povidone-iodine or alcohol swab. Attach the secondary infusion set to the Y-site and secure it. Adjust each infusion rate independently. Remember that with this setup, you don't have a backcheck valve above the Y-site, so one solution may flow back into the other.

Giving I.V. therapy to elderly patients
I.V. therapy for elderly patients poses special nursing challenges, especially regarding the effects of age-related differences in the skin and veins on I.V. line insertion and maintenance. Be sure to check with your state board of licensing for individual guidelines regarding the specific restrictions for LPN's and I.V. therapy.

Because an elderly person's veins are usually more prominent and his skin is less resistant, you may find venipuncture easier than in children. Even so, the normal aging process also presents drawbacks. Because the tissues are looser, you may have more difficulty stabilizing the vein. Also, because veins become more fragile, you'll need to perform the venipuncture quickly and efficiently to avoid excessive bruising. A smaller gauge needle, such as a 24G ¾" needle, may be more appropriate and easier to insert. You'll also need to remove the tourniquet promptly to prevent increased vascular pressure from causing bleeding through the vein wall around the infusion device.

Typically, an elderly patient's veins appears full of twists and turns because of the skin's increased transparency and decreased elasticity. They'll also appear large if venous pressure is adequate. Winged steel needles may be used as I.V. insertion devices for elderly patients because they are less thrombogenic, can be easily manipulated, and lie flat against the skin to provide a stable site for the device. However, these needles increase the risk of infiltration.

To help stabilize the vein for insertion, stretch the skin around the insertion site and anchor it firmly with your nondominant hand. Smaller, shorter access devices usually work best with an elderly patient's fragile veins.

Complications of I.V. therapy

Complications of peripheral I.V. therapy can arise from the access device, the infusion, or the drug being administered and can be local or systemic.

Local complications include:
- infiltration
- phlebitis
- catheter dislodgment
- occlusion
- vein irritation or pain at the I.V. site
- severed or fractured catheter
- hematoma
- venous spasm
- vasovagal reaction
- thrombosis
- thrombophlebitis
- nerve, tendon, or ligament damage.

Systemic complications include air embolism and allergic reaction. A complication may begin locally and become systemic — as when an infection at the venipuncture site progresses to septicemia. (For a complete description see *Local and systemic complications of peripheral I.V. therapy,* pages 76 to 85.)

INFILTRATION

Perhaps the greatest threat to a patient receiving I.V. therapy is *infiltration,* or infused fluid leaking into the surrounding tissues. Infiltra-

> **DOCUMENTATION TIPS**
>
> ## Documenting complications
>
> If complications occur, document:
> - signs and symptoms
> - patient complaints
> - name of the physician notified, and treatment.
>
> For example, if your patient develops a severe infusion-related problem — vesicant infiltration, circulatory compromise, fluid overload, a skin tear, or severe allergic reaction — fill out an incident report according to your facility's policy and procedures. For legal purposes, document the details of the complication as well as medical and nursing interventions.

tion occurs when the access device punctures the vein wall or migrates out of the vein. The risk of infiltration may be as much as 70% greater with a steel needle than with a plastic catheter, depending on the skill of the person performing the venipuncture and the patient's compliance.

Infiltration involving steel needles can occur any time after starting an infusion. With plastic catheters, infiltration is more likely to occur after a day or more, usually because the flexible tip of the catheter has penetrated the vein wall.

With either venipuncture device, the risk of infiltration increases whenever you insert it near a joint. If the tip of the venipuncture device isn't inserted far enough into the vein lumen, part of the tip remains outside the vein and infiltration develops quickly.

Infiltration of a drug or solution can result in extravasation and breakdown of tissue (necrosis) if the drug or solution is a vesicant.

The type of fluid being infused determines how much discomfort the patient feels during infiltration. Isotonic fluids usually don't cause much discomfort. Fluids with an acidic or alkaline pH, or those that are more than slightly hypertonic, are usually more irritating. Don't depend on the patient to complain of discomfort; large amounts of I.V. fluid — as much as 1 L — can escape into the surrounding tissues without the patient knowing it.

Fortunately, you can minimize or prevent most complications by using proper insertion techniques and carefully monitoring the patient. I.V. sites should be checked by a nurse every 2 to 4 hours, or according to facility policy. If complications do occur, don't forget to document them. (See *Documenting complications*.)

(Text continues on page 84.)

Local and systemic complications of peripheral I.V. therapy

Complications of peripheral I.V. therapy may be local or systemic. These tables list some common complications along with their signs and symptoms, causes, and nursing interventions, including preventive measures.

SIGNS AND SYMPTOMS	CAUSES
LOCAL COMPLICATIONS	
PHLEBITIS • Tenderness at tip of device and above • Redness at tip of catheter and along vein • Puffy area over vein • Vein hard on palpation • Elevated temperature	• Poor blood flow around device • Friction from catheter movement in vein • Device left in vein too long • Clotting at catheter tip (thrombophlebitis) • Solution with high or low pH or high osmolarity
INFILTRATION • Swelling at and around I.V. site (may extend along entire limb) • Discomfort, burning, or pain at site • Feeling of tightness at site • Decreased skin temperature around site • Blanching at site • Continuing fluid infusion even when vein is occluded, although rate may decrease • Absent backflow of blood • Slower flow rate	• Device dislodged from vein or perforated vein
CATHETER DISLODGMENT • Catheter partly backed out of vein • Infusate infiltrating	• Loosened tape or tubing snagged in bedclothes, resulting in partial retraction of catheter

Nursing interventions

- Remove the device.
- Apply a warm pack.
- Notify the physician.
- Document the patient's condition and your interventions.
  Prevention:
- Restart the infusion using a larger vein for irritating infusate, or restart with a smaller-gauge device to ensure adequate blood flow.
- Tape device securely to prevent motion.

- Remove the device.
- Apply warm soaks to aid absorption.
- Elevate the limb.
- If severe, notify the physician.
- Periodically assess circulation by checking for pulse, capillary refill, and numbness or tingling.
- Restart the infusion, preferably in another limb or above the infiltration site.
- Document the patient's condition and your interventions.
  Prevention:
- Check the I.V. site frequently, especially when using an I.V. pump.
- Don't obscure area above site with tape.
- Teach the patient to report discomfort, pain, or swelling.

- If no infiltration occurs, retape without pushing catheter back into vein.
  Prevention:
- Tape the device securely on insertion.

(continued)

Local and systemic complications of peripheral I.V. therapy *(continued)*

SIGNS AND SYMPTOMS	CAUSES
LOCAL COMPLICATIONS *(continued)*	
OCCLUSION • No increase in flow rate when I.V. container is raised • Blood backup in line • Discomfort at insertion site	• I.V. flow interrupted • Intermittent device not flushed • Blood backup in line when patient walks • Hypercoagulable patient • Line clamped too long
VEIN IRRITATION OR PAIN AT I.V. SITE • Pain during infusion • Possible blanching if vasospasm occurs • Red skin over vein during infusion • Rapidly developing signs of phlebitis	• Solution with high or low pH or high osmolarity, such as potassium chloride, phenytoin, and some antibiotics (vancomycin and nafcillin)
SEVERED CATHETER • Leakage from catheter shaft	• Catheter inadvertently cut by scissors • Reinsertion of needle into catheter
HEMATOMA • Tenderness at venipuncture site • Bruising around site • Inability to advance or flush I.V. line	• Vein punctured through ventral wall at time of venipuncture • Leakage of blood from needle displacement

Complications of I.V. therapy ■ 79

NURSING INTERVENTIONS

- Use a low flush pressure syringe during injection. Don't use force. If resistance is met, stop immediately. If unsuccessful, reinsert the I.V. device.
  Prevention:
- Maintain the I.V. flow rate.
- Flush promptly after intermittent piggyback administration.
- Have the patient walk with his arm below heart level to reduce the risk of blood back-up.

- Slow the flow rate.
- Try using an electronic-flow device to achieve a steady regulated flow.
  Prevention:
- Dilute solutions before administration. For example, give antibiotics in 250-ml rather than 100-ml solution. If the drug has a low pH, ask the pharmacist if the drug can be buffered with sodium bicarbonate. (Refer to facility policy.)
- If long-term therapy is planned, ask the physician to use central I.V. line.

- If the broken part is visible, try to retrieve it. If unsuccessful, notify the physician.
- If a portion of the catheter enters the bloodstream, place a tourniquet above the I.V. site to prevent progression.
- Notify the physician and radiology.
- Document the patient's condition and your interventions.
  Prevention:
- Don't use scissors around the I.V. site.
- Never reinsert a needle into catheter.
- Remove the unsuccessfully inserted catheter and needle together.

- Remove the infusion device.
- Apply pressure and warm soaks to the affected area.
- Recheck for bleeding.
- Document the patient's condition and your interventions.
  Prevention:
- Choose a vein that can accommodate the size of the intended device.
- Release the tourniquet as soon as successful insertion is achieved.

(continued)

Local and systemic complications of peripheral I.V. therapy *(continued)*

SIGNS AND SYMPTOMS	CAUSES
LOCAL COMPLICATIONS *(continued)*	
VENOUS SPASM • Pain along vein • Sluggish infusion rate when clamp is completely open • Blanched skin over vein	• Severe vein irritation from irritating drugs or fluids • Administration of cold fluids or blood • Very rapid flow rate (with fluids at room temperature)
THROMBOSIS • Painful, reddened, and swollen vein • Sluggish or stopped I.V. flow	• Injury to endothelial cells of vein wall, allowing platelets to adhere and thrombus to form
THROMBOPHLEBITIS • Severe discomfort • Reddened, swollen, and hardened vein	• Thrombosis and inflammation
NERVE, TENDON, OR LIGAMENT DAMAGE • Extreme pain (similar to electric shock when nerve is contracted) • Numbness and muscle contraction • Delayed effects, including paralysis, numbness, and deformity	• Improper venipuncture technique, resulting in injury to surrounding nerves, tendons, or ligaments • Tight taping or improper splinting with arm board

Nursing interventions

- Apply warm soaks over the vein and surrounding area.
- Slow the infusion rate.
  Prevention:
- Use blood warmer for blood or packed red blood cells when appropriate.

- Remove the device; restart the infusion in the opposite limb if possible.
- Apply warm soaks.
- Watch for I.V. therapy-related infection. (Thrombi provide an excellent environment for bacterial growth.)
- If infusion rate is sluggish, don't try to irrigate the line. This could increase the risk of infection or flush a clot into the bloodstream, resulting in an embolus.
  Prevention:
- Use proper venipuncture techniques to reduce injury to the vein.

- Remove the device; restart the infusion in the opposite limb if possible.
- Apply warm soaks.
- Notify the physician.
- Watch for I.V. therapy-related infection. (Thrombi provide an excellent environment for bacterial growth.)
  Prevention:
- Check the site frequently. Remove the device at the first sign of redness and tenderness.

- Stop the procedure and remove the device.
  Prevention:
- Don't repeatedly penetrate tissues with the venous access device.
- Don't apply excessive pressure when taping or encircle the limb with tape.
- Pad the arm board and, if possible, pad the tape securing the arm board.

(continued)

Local and systemic complications of peripheral I.V. therapy (continued)

SIGNS AND SYMPTOMS	CAUSES
SYSTEMIC COMPLICATIONS	
CIRCULATORY OVERLOAD ● Discomfort ● Jugular vein engorgement ● Respiratory distress ● Increased blood pressure ● Crackles ● Large positive fluid balance (intake is greater than output)	● Roller clamp loosened to allow run-on infusion ● Flow rate too rapid ● Miscalculation of fluid requirements
SYSTEMIC INFECTION (SEPTICEMIA OR BACTEREMIA) ● Fever, chills, and malaise for no apparent reason ● Changes in blood pressure ● Contaminated I.V. site, usually with no visible signs of infection at site	● Failure to maintain aseptic technique during insertion or site care ● Severe phlebitis, which can set up ideal conditions for organism growth ● Poor taping that permits infusion device to move, which can introduce organisms into bloodstream ● Prolonged indwelling time of device ● Immunocompromised patient
AIR EMBOLISM ● Respiratory distress ● Unequal breath sounds ● Weak pulse ● Increased central venous pressure ● Decreased blood pressure ● Confusion, disorientation, loss of consciousness	● Empty solution container ● Solution container empties; next container pushes air down line ● Tubing disconnected from venous access device or I.V. bag

Nursing interventions

- Raise the head of the bed.
- Slow the infusion rate (but don't remove the venous access device).
- Administer oxygen as needed.
- Notify the physician.
- Give ordered drugs (probably furosemide).
- Monitor input and output.
- Keep patient warm to promote peripheral circulation.
  Prevention:
- Use a pump, volume-control set, controller, or rate minder for elderly or compromised patients.
- Recheck calculations of fluid requirements.
- Monitor the infusion frequently.

- Notify the physician.
- Give ordered drugs.
- Culture the site and the device.
- Monitor the patent's vital signs.
  Prevention:
- Use aseptic technique when handling solutions and tubings, inserting the venous access device, and discontinuing the infusion.
- Secure all connections.
- Change I.V. solutions, tubing, and venous access device at recommended times.
- Use I.V. filters.

- Stop the infusion.
- Place the patient in Trendelenburg's position on his left side to allow air to enter the right atrium and disperse through the pulmonary artery.
- Administer oxygen.
- Notify the physician.
- Document the patient's condition and your interventions.
  Prevention:
- Purge the tubing of air completely before the infusion.
- Use an air-detection device on the pump or an air-eliminating filter close to the I.V. site.

(continued)

Local and systemic complications of peripheral I.V. therapy *(continued)*

SIGNS AND SYMPTOMS	CAUSES

SYSTEMIC COMPLICATIONS *(continued)*

ALLERGIC REACTION
- Itching
- Tearing eyes and runny nose
- Bronchospasm
- Wheezing
- Urticarial rash
- Edema at I.V. site

- Allergy to drug or other allergens

Stopping I.V. therapy

To stop the infusion, first clamp the infusion line; then remove the venipuncture device using aseptic technique. Here's how to proceed:
- After putting on gloves, lift the tape from the skin to expose the insertion site. You don't need to remove the tape or dressing as long as you can peel it back to expose the venipuncture device and skin.
- Don't manipulate the device in the skin to prevent skin organisms from entering the bloodstream. Moving the device may also cause discomfort, especially if the insertion site has become phlebitic.
- Apply a sterile 2″ × 2″ dressing directly over the insertion site; then quickly remove the device.

RED FLAG Never use an alcohol pad to clean the site when stopping an infusion; this may cause bleeding and a burning sensation.

- Maintain direct pressure on the I.V. site for several minutes, then tape a dressing over it, being careful not to encircle the limb. If

NURSING INTERVENTIONS

- Secure all connections.
- If a reaction occurs, stop the infusion immediately and infuse normal saline solution.
- Maintain a patent airway.
- Notify the physician.
- Give an antihistaminic steroid, an antiinflammatory, or an antipyretic.
- Give 0.2 to 0.5 ml of 1:1,000 aqueous epinephrine subcutaneously. Repeat at 3-minute intervals and as needed and ordered.
- Administer ordered cortisone.
  Prevention:
- Obtain the patient's allergy history. Be aware of cross-allergies.
- Assist with test dosing.
- Monitor the patient carefully during the first 15 minutes of receiving a new drug.

possible, hold the limb upright for about 5 minutes to decrease venous pressure.
- Tell the patient to restrict his activity for about 10 minutes and to leave the site dressing in place for at least 8 hours. If he feels lingering tenderness at the I.V. site, apply warm, moist packs.
- Dispose of the used venipuncture equipment, tubing, and solution containers in a receptacle designated by your facility.
- Document the time of removal, the catheter length and integrity, and the condition of the site. Also, record how the patient tolerated the procedure and any nursing interventions.

3

CENTRAL VENOUS THERAPY

Understanding central venous therapy

In central venous (CV) therapy, drugs or fluids are infused directly into a major vein. CV therapy is used in various situations, including when a patient requires emergency care or when a patient's peripheral veins are inaccessible. It may also be ordered when a patient needs:
- an infusion of a large volume of fluid
- multiple infusions
- long-term venous therapy
- an infusion of irritating drugs such as potassium
- an infusion of fluids with high osmolarity such as total parenteral nutrition (TPN).

At one time, only patients in intensive care and specialty units received CV therapy. Today, patients in any unit or even at home may receive CV therapy.

BENEFITS
Benefits of CV therapy include:
- access to the central veins
- rapid infusion of drugs or large amounts of fluids
- a way to draw blood samples and measure CV pressure, an important indicator of circulatory function
- reduced need for repeated venipunctures, which decreases the patient's anxiety and preserves (or restores) the peripheral veins
- reduced risk of vein irritation from infusing irritating or caustic drugs.

RISKS
Like any other invasive procedure, CV therapy has its drawbacks. It increases the risk of such life-threatening complications as:
- pneumothorax
- sepsis
- thrombus formation
- perforation of the vessel and adjacent organs.

Using a CV catheter also has disadvantages:
- It requires more time and skill to insert than a peripheral I.V. catheter.
- It costs more to maintain than a peripheral I.V. catheter.
- It carries a risk of air embolism.

VENOUS CIRCULATION
The 5 L of blood in an average adult moves throughout the entire body. After delivering oxygen and nutrients throughout the body, depleted blood flows from the capillaries to wider and wider veins and finally returns to the right side of the heart before collecting a fresh supply of oxygen from the lungs. CV circulation enters the right atrium through two major veins: the superior and inferior vena cava.

Before flowing into the right atrium, venous return from the head, neck, and arms enters the superior vena cava through three main routes:
- internal and external jugular veins
- subclavian vein
- right and left innominate veins.

Venous return from the legs enters the inferior vena cava and returns blood to the right atrium through several routes, including the femoral venous system and multiple accessory venous pathways throughout the abdomen.

In CV therapy, the tip of a catheter is inserted in one of two places: the superior vena cava and inferior vena cava. Where the catheter goes depends on which veins are accessible and which type of infusion is ordered.

Blood flows unimpeded around the tip at about 2,000 ml/minute, allowing a rapid infusion of large amounts of fluid directly into the circulation. Because fluids are rapidly diluted by the venous circulation, highly concentrated or caustic fluids can be infused. (See *CV catheter pathways,* pages 88 and 89.)

In a variation of CV therapy, a catheter is inserted through a peripheral vein and the catheter tip is passed all the way to the superior vena cava. For instance, a catheter inserted in the arm (at the an-

CV catheter pathways

Usually, a central venous (CV) catheter is inserted into the subclavian vein or the internal jugular vein. The catheter should terminate in the superior vena cava. The illustrations below show several common pathways for a CV catheter.

Inserted into the subclavian vein, this CV catheter terminates in the superior vena cava.

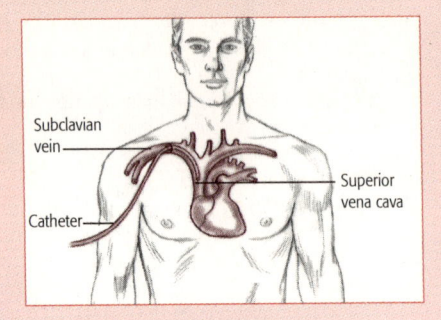

This CV catheter, peripherally inserted into the basilic vein, terminates in the superior vena cava.

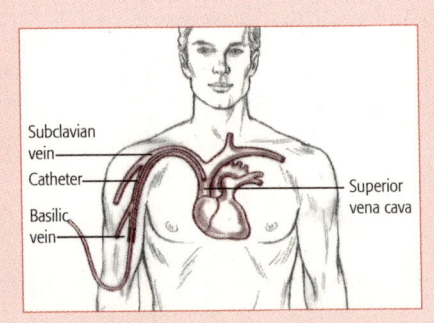

tecubital fossa) enters the basilic vein and is threaded through the subclavian and brachiocephalic veins to the superior vena cava. To ease this procedure, newer catheters have longer introducers, smaller lumens, and variable lengths.

LIFE STAGES Because children are smaller, they require a shorter catheter with a smaller lumen than adults.

TYPES OF CENTRAL VENOUS CATHETERS
You may see these types of CV catheters in use:
- nontunneled catheters

Understanding central venous therapy ■ 89

This CV catheter enters the internal jugular vein and terminates in the superior vena cava.

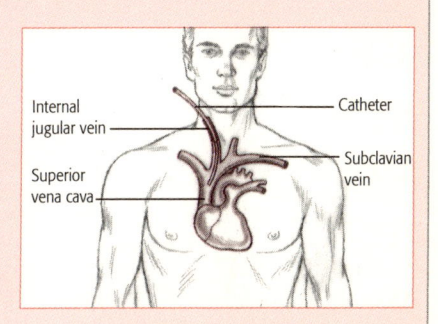

This CV catheter enters the subclavian vein and terminates in the superior vena cava. Note that the catheter tunnels (shown by broken line) from the insertion site, through the subcutaneous tissue, to an exit site on the skin (usually located by the nipple). Also note how the position of the Dacron cuff helps hold the catheter in place.

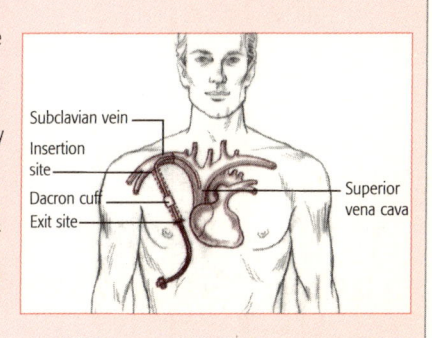

- tunneled catheters
- peripherally inserted central catheters (PICCs)
- implanted vascular access ports (VAPs).

Selecting the appropriate CV catheter for a patient depends on the type of therapy needed.

Nontunneled

Nontunneled catheters, also called central catheters, are radiopaque, so placement can be checked by X-ray. They're usually designed for short-term use, such as brief continuation of I.V. therapy after a patient has been in the hospital, and may not be appropriate for a patient starting long-term I.V. therapy.

To avoid infection, nontunneled catheters are changed according to facility's policy. The optimal time interval for using this catheter is unknown; the insertion site must be frequently monitored. If the injection site appears red or if infection is suspected, the access site shouldn't be used and an alternative site should be found. Signs and symptoms of infection should be reported to the physician.

Tunneled

Tunneled CV catheters are designed for long-term use. They're also radiopaque and usually made of silicone. Silicone is much less likely to cause thrombosis than polyurethane and polyvinyl chloride are because silicone is more physiologically compatible. This minimizes irritation or damage to the vein lining.

A tunneled CV catheter has a cuff that encourages tissue growth within the tunnel. In about 1 week, the tissue anchors the catheter in place and keeps bacteria out of venous circulation. In most cases, the cuff is made of polyethylene terephthalate fiber. Another type of cuff contains silver ions that provide antibacterial protection for about 3 months.

Tunneled catheters are better suited to the home-care patient than nontunneled catheters. They're also used in patients who have poor peripheral venous access or need long-term daily infusions and who have:
- cancer
- acquired immunodeficiency syndrome (AIDS)
- intestinal malabsorption
- anemia
- bone or organ infections
- other chronic diseases.

Drugs that are given by a tunneled CV catheter include:
- antibiotics
- chemotherapy
- TPN
- blood products.

TUNNELED TYPES

Common tunneled catheters for long-term use include the Broviac, Hickman, and Groshong catheters. Tunneled catheters can be single-lumen, double-lumen, triple-lumen, or multi-lumen and can vary in size. The Broviac tunneled CV catheter is a good choice for a patient — such as a child — with small central veins. (See *Guide to CV catheters,* pages 92 to 97.)

Peripherally inserted central catheters

The most commonly used catheter for peripheral CV therapy is the PICC. A PICC, also known as a long-arm or long-line catheter, is inserted through a peripheral vein, with the tip ending in the superior vena cava. If the catheter tip is located outside the vena cava, it's no longer considered a central catheter and should be removed.

Generally, PICCs are used when patients need infusions of caustic drugs (such as long-term antibiotic therapy) or solutions. They're also used in patients who need transfusions. PICCs are especially useful if the patient doesn't have a reliable route for short-term I.V. therapy.

When a patient needs CV therapy for 5 days to several months or requires repeated venous access, a PICC may be the best choice. A PICC may also be ordered when a patient has a chest injury from trauma or burns or respiratory problems due to chronic obstructive pulmonary disease (COPD), or other conditions. Using a peripheral insertion site for a PICC helps prevent complications such as pneumothorax that may occur with a CV line.

PICCs are commonly used in patients with such conditions as:
- AIDS
- cancer
- recurrent infections (such as osteomyelitis and endocarditis)
- sickle cell anemia
- women who require I.V. therapy due to severe morning sickness.

Infusions commonly given by PICC include:
- analgesics
- antibiotics
- blood products
- chemotherapy
- immunoglobulins
- opioids
- TPN.

PICCs are available with a single or double lumen and with or without guide wires. A guide wire stiffens the catheter to ease its advancement through the vein, but it can damage the vein if used incorrectly.

The patient receiving PICC therapy must have a peripheral vein large enough to accept an introducer needle. Catheter gauge depends on the size of the patient's vein and the type of fluid or drug to be infused. PICCs range from 14G to 24G in diameter and from

Guide to CV catheters

Central venous (CV) catheters differ in their design, composition, and indications for use. This chart outlines the advantages, disadvantages, and nursing considerations for several commonly used catheters.

CATHETER DESCRIPTION AND INDICATIONS	ADVANTAGES AND DISADVANTAGES

SHORT-TERM, SINGLE-LUMEN CATHETER

DESCRIPTION
- Polyurethane or silicone rubber
- Approximately 8" (20 cm) long
- Variety of lumen gauges

INDICATIONS
- Short-term CV access
- Emergency access
- When only a single lumen is required

ADVANTAGES
- Can be inserted at bedside
- Easily removed
- Stiffness aids central venous pressure (CVP) monitoring

DISADVANTAGES
- Has limited functions
- Should be changed every 3 to 7 days (depending on facility policy).

SHORT-TERM, MULTILUMEN CATHETER

DESCRIPTION
- Polyurethane or silicone rubber
- Double, triple, or quadruple lumen at 3/4" (1.9 cm) intervals
- Variety of lumen gauges

INDICATIONS
- Short-term CV access
- Limited insertion sites when multiple infusions are required

ADVANTAGES
- Can be inserted at bedside
- Easily removed
- Stiffness aids CVP monitoring
- Allows infusion of multiple solutions through the same catheter — even for the same task (for example, incompatible solutions)

DISADVANTAGES
- Limited functions
- Needs to be changed every 3 to 7 days

---

7 3/4" to 23 1/2" (20 to 60 cm) in length. Other PICCs are configured for use in a neonate. If the patient will receive blood or blood products through the PICC, at least an 18G catheter is used. (See *Guide to PICCs*, pages 98 and 99.)

A tuberculin syringe or a 3-ml syringe isn't used with a PICC to give a drug or flush a catheter. These syringes create too much pressure (measured in pounds per square inch) in the line. Such excessive pressure can cause the device to burst. The appropriate syringe size is 10 ml.

NURSING CONSIDERATIONS

- Assess frequently for signs of infection and clot formation.

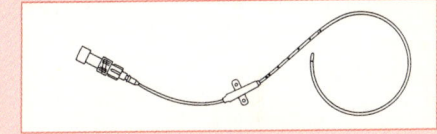

- Know the gauge and purpose of each lumen.
- The same lumen is used for the same task (for example, to administer total parenteral nutrition or to collect a blood sample).

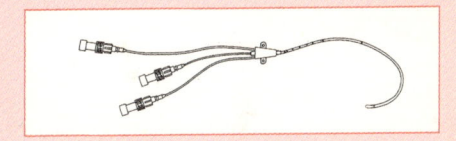

(continued)

In many states, the nurse practice act allows registered nurses (RNs) who are trained and skilled in the proper technique to insert PICCs. PICCs are widely used for home infusion therapy because they may be inserted at the bedside without a physician in attendance.

The term PICC may be incorrectly used to describe an extended peripheral catheter. This catheter is more correctly known as a midline device. Technically, the midline device isn't a CV catheter

(Text continues on page 96.)

Guide to CV catheters (continued)

CATHETER DESCRIPTION AND INDICATIONS	ADVANTAGES AND DISADVANTAGES

GROSHONG CATHETER

DESCRIPTION
- Silicone rubber
- About 35" (88.9 cm) long
- Closed end with pressure-sensitive two-way valve
- Dacron cuff
- Available with single or double lumen
- Tunneled

INDICATIONS
- Long-term CV access
- Heparin allergy

ADVANTAGES
- Thrombosis is less likely than with catheters made with polyvinyl chloride.
- Pressure-sensitive two- and three-way valve eliminates heparin flushes.
- Polyethylene terephthalate fiber cuff anchors catheter and prevents bacterial migration.

DISADVANTAGES
- Requires surgical insertion
- Tears and kinks easily
- Difficult to clear substances from its tip because of blunt end

HICKMAN CATHETER

DESCRIPTION
- Silicone rubber
- About 35" long
- Open end with clamp
- Polyethylene terephthalate fiber cuff 11¾" (29.9 cm) from hub
- Tunneled

INDICATIONS
- Long-term CV access
- Home therapy

ADVANTAGES
- Polyethylene terephthalate fiber cuff prevents excess motion and organism migration.
- Clamps eliminate need for the Valsalva maneuver.

DISADVANTAGES
- Requires surgical insertion
- Has an open end
- Requires a physician for removal
- Tears and kinks easily

BROVIAC CATHETER

DESCRIPTION
- Silicone rubber
- About 35" long
- Open end with clamp
- Polyethylene terephthalate fiber cuff 11³/₄" from hub
- Tunneled

INDICATIONS
- Long-term CV access
- Small central vessels, such as pediatric or elderly patients

ADVANTAGES
- Small lumen more comfortable

DISADVANTAGES
- Small lumen limits use
- Can't infuse multiple solutions at once
- In children, growth may cause the catheter tip to move its position outside the superior vena cava

Understanding central venous therapy

NURSING CONSIDERATIONS

- Two surgical sites require dressing after insertion.
- Handle the catheter gently.
- Check the external portion frequently for kinks or leaks. (Repair kit is available.)
- Observe frequently for kinks or tears.
- The lumen needs to be flushed with enough saline solution to clear the catheter, especially after drawing or administering blood.
- The end caps are changed weekly.

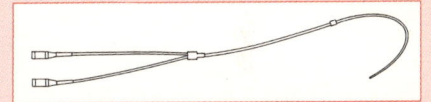

- Two surgical sites require dressing after insertion.
- Handle the catheter gently.
- Observe frequently for kinks or tears. (Repair kit is available.)
- Clamp the catheter whenever it becomes disconnected or open, using a clamp on the catheter.
- The catheter is flushed daily when not in use per manufacturer's guidelines.

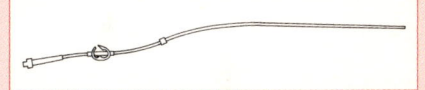

- Drawing or administering of blood products must be done according to facility policy.
- The catheter is flushed daily when not in use and before and after each use per facility policy.

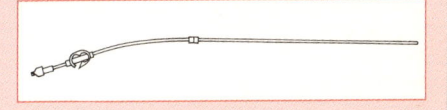

(continued)

Guide to CV catheters (continued)

CATHETER DESCRIPTION AND INDICATIONS	ADVANTAGES AND DISADVANTAGES
HICKMAN-BROVIAC CATHETER	
DESCRIPTION • Hickman and Broviac catheters combined in one catheter *INDICATIONS* • Long-term CV access • When multiple infusions are required	*ADVANTAGES* • Double-lumen Hickman catheter for sampling and administration of blood • Broviac lumen for I.V. fluids, including TPN fluids *DISADVANTAGES* • Requires surgical insertion • Has an open end • Requires a physician for removal • Tears and kinks easily
LONG-LINE CATHETER	
DESCRIPTION • Peripherally inserted central catheter • Silicone rubber • 20" to 24" (51 to 61 cm) long; available in 14G, 16G, 18G, 20G, 22G, and 24G *INDICATIONS* • Long-term CV access • Poor central access • High risk for complications from insertion at central access sites • When patient will have or has had head and neck surgery	*ADVANTAGES* • Peripherally inserted • Can be inserted at bedside with minimal complications • May be inserted by a trained registered nurse in most states • Single lumen or double lumen *DISADVANTAGES* • May occlude smaller peripheral vessels • May be difficult to keep immobile

because its tip doesn't rest in the CV circulation but in the axillary vein.

A true PICC tip terminates in the superior or inferior vena cava. When caring for a patient with a PICC, make sure you know where the catheter terminates and the entire length of the catheter, both indwelling and external.

ADVANTAGES
PICCs have definite advantages over other forms of central lines:

Nursing considerations

- The lumens are labeled to prevent confusion.
- When not in use, the catheter is flushed, and before and after each use, per facility policy.

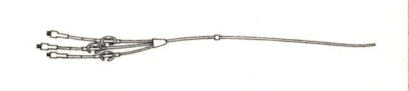

- Check frequently for signs of phlebitis and thrombus formation.
- The catheter is inserted above the antecubital fossa.
- Use an arm board if necessary.
- The catheter may alter CVP measurements.

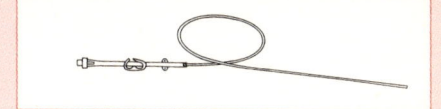

- They provide long-term access to central veins. A PICC can be left in place for long periods (unless complications develop) because the catheter is made of soft, physiologically compatible silicone or polyurethane. A single catheter may be used for an entire course of therapy.
- They provide a safe, reliable route for infusion therapy and occasional blood sampling.

(Text continues on page 100.)

Guide to PICCs

Here are some of the peripherally inserted central catheters (PICCs) that are currently available.

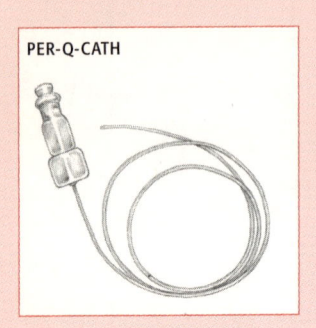

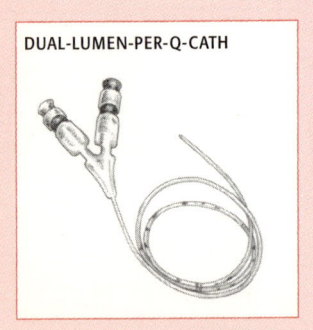

PER-Q-CATH

DUAL-LUMEN-PER-Q-CATH

Per-Q-Cath and Dual-Lumen Per-Q-Cath are manufactured by Bard Access Systems. Features include:
- single lumen or double lumen
- gauges from 16G to 23G
- catheter length of 23" (58 cm)
- insertion tray available
- repair kit available.

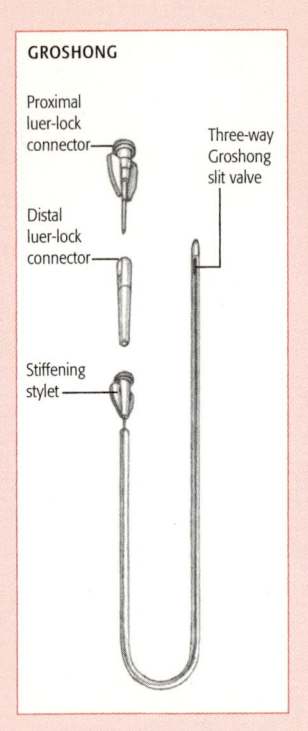

GROSHONG

Proximal luer-lock connector

Three-way Groshong slit valve

Distal luer-lock connector

Stiffening stylet

Groshong is manufactured by Bard Access Systems. Features include:
- single lumen or double lumen
- gauges from 18G to 20G
- catheter lengths from 22½" to 23" (57 to 58 cm).

Understanding central venous therapy ■ 99

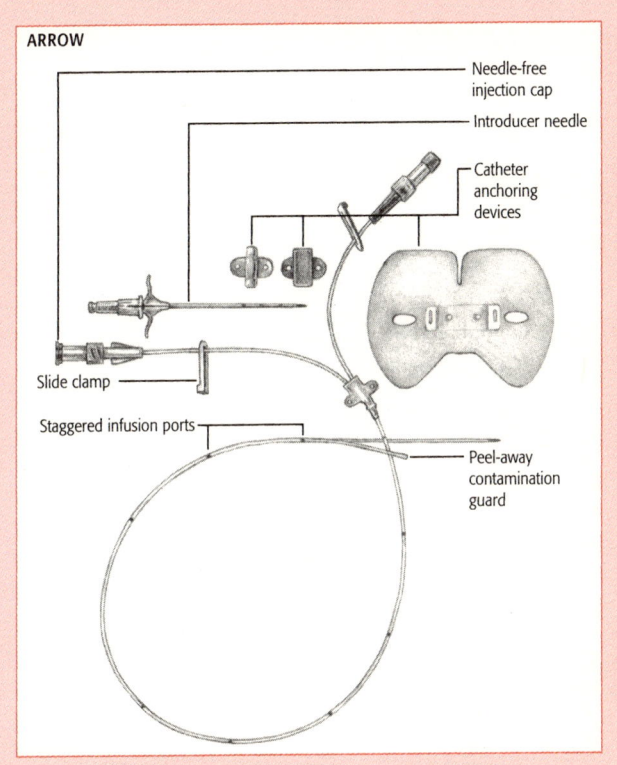

ARROW

- Needle-free injection cap
- Introducer needle
- Catheter anchoring devices
- Slide clamp
- Staggered infusion ports
- Peel-away contamination guard

Arrow is manufactured by Arrow International. Features include:
- single lumen or double lumen
- gauges from 18G to 20G
- polyurethane or silicone rubber catheter
- stylet-free insertion
- peel-away guard to maintain catheter sterility during insertion
- tip that deflects on contact with vessel walls to reduce irritation during insertion
- anchoring device available on some.

Comparing VAPs to long-term CV catheters

A vascular access port (VAP) offers the patient many of the advantages of a long-term central venous (CV) catheter, along with an unobtrusive design that many patients find easier to accept. Both devices are indicated when poor venous access prohibits peripheral I.V. therapy. Which device is most appropriate to use depends on the type and duration of treatment, the frequency of access, and the patient's condition. This table compares and contrasts the two devices.

	VAP	**LONG-TERM CATHETER**
THERAPY TYPE		
Continuous infusion of drugs or fluids	Yes, but maintaining continuous needle access eliminates the benefits of implantation	Yes
Self-administration of drugs or fluids	Yes, but it may be more difficult for the patient or family member to manage	Yes
Bolus injections of vesicant or irritant drugs by health care professionals	Yes	Yes

- They minimize the risk of blood clots and phlebitis associated with other types of CV catheters.
- They're extremely cost-effective compared with other long- and short-term CV catheters.

DISADVANTAGES
A PICC may be unsuitable for a patient with bruises, scarring, or sclerosis from earlier multiple venipunctures at the intended PICC site. Bedside ultrasound may be used to assess whether a vein is suitable for a PICC. Keep in mind that a PICC works best when it's introduced early in treatment; it shouldn't be considered as a last resort.

Implanted vascular access ports
As the number of chronically ill patients increases, so does the need for long-term I.V. therapy. When an external catheter isn't suitable, an implanted device may be used.

Comparing VAPs to long-term CV catheters
(continued)

	VAP	**LONG-TERM CATHETER**
THERAPY LENGTH		
Less than 3 months	No, because the high cost of implanting and removing the device precludes it	Yes
More than 3 months	Yes, but the cost of implantation and removal may exceed the cost benefit if treatment lasts less than 6 months	Yes
ACCESS FREQUENCY		
Three or more times per week	Yes, but it may minimize the advantage of having an implanted device	Yes
Less than once per week	Yes	No, because the high cost of maintaining the catheter precludes it
PATIENT CONCERNS		
Negative effect on body image	No	Possibly
Negative reaction to needle punctures	Possibly	No
Ability to care for external catheter	Not needed	Needed
Cost of dressing changes and heparinization	Minimal	Considerable

An implanted VAP functions much like a long-term CV catheter except that it has no external parts; it's implanted in a pocket under the skin. (See *Comparing VAPs to long-term CV catheters.*)

Understanding implantable pumps

An implantable pump is usually placed in a subcutaneous pocket made in the abdomen below the umbilicus. An implantable pump has two chambers separated by a bellows. One chamber contains the I.V. solution; the other contains a charging fluid. The charging fluid chamber exerts continuous pressure on the bellows, forcing the infusion solution through the silicone outlet catheter into a central vein. The pump also has an auxiliary septum that can be used for bolus injections. Generally, the pump is indicated for patients who require continuous low-volume infusions.

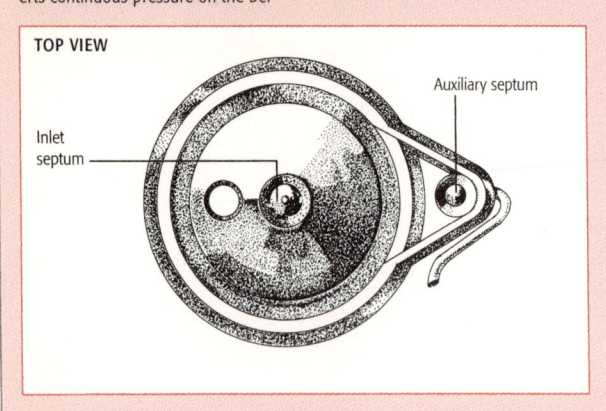

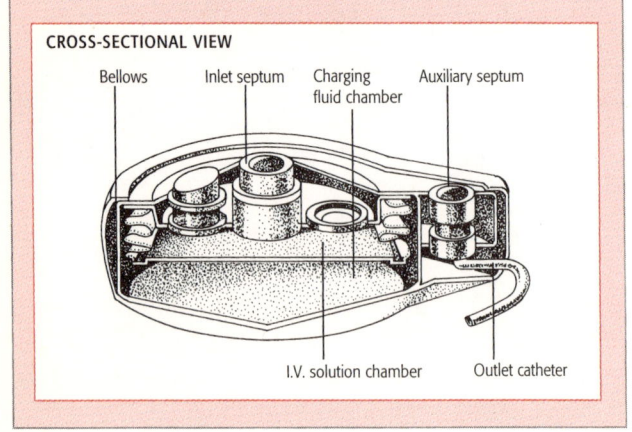

TOP VIEW

- Inlet septum
- Auxiliary septum

CROSS-SECTIONAL VIEW

- Bellows
- Inlet septum
- Charging fluid chamber
- Auxiliary septum
- I.V. solution chamber
- Outlet catheter

The indwelling catheter that's attached to a VAP is surgically tunneled under the skin until the catheter tip lies in the superior vena cava. The catheter may be threaded through the subclavian vein at the shoulder or through the jugular vein at the base of the neck, for example. A VAP is also suitable for epidural, intra-arterial, or intraperitoneal placement.

ADVANTAGES

Implanted devices are easier to maintain than external devices. They need to be heparinized only once a month to maintain patency. VAPs also pose less risk of infection because they have no exit site through which microorganisms can invade. VAPs offer several other advantages for patients, including:
- minimal activity restrictions
- few self-care measures for the patient to learn and perform
- few dressing changes (except when accessed and used to maintain continuous infusions or intermittent infusion devices).

Finally, because VAPs create only a slight protrusion under the skin, many patients find them easier to accept than external venous access devices. A patient with a VAP may shower, swim, and exercise without worrying about the device, as long as the device isn't accessed. The physician decides how soon after insertion the patient may undertake these activities.

DISADVANTAGES

Because it's implanted, a VAP may be more difficult for a patient to manage, especially for daily or frequent infusions. Accessing the device requires insertion of a specialized needle through subcutaneous tissue, which may be uncomfortable for patients who fear or dislike needle punctures.

Implanting and removing the VAP requires surgery and possible hospitalization, which can be costly. The comparatively high cost of a VAP makes it worthwhile only for patients who require infusion therapy for at least 6 months. Another type of implantable vascular access device — for example, an implantable pump — may be used for patients who require continuous low-volume infusions. (See *Understanding implantable pumps*.)

Preparing for central venous therapy

To prepare for CV therapy, an insertion site for the CV catheter must be selected. You may then prepare the patient both physically and mentally for the insertion procedure. Before the procedure, gather and prepare the appropriate equipment.

SELECTING THE INSERTION SITE

LIFE STAGES *In infants, the jugular vein is the preferred insertion site, even though it's much more difficult to maintain than other sites. Usually the physician and the patient's family select a mutually acceptable site if the catheter will be used for long-term therapy.*

With the exception of PICC insertions, CV devices are usually inserted by a physician.

In CV therapy, the insertion site depends on these variables:
- type of catheter
- patient's anatomy and age
- duration of therapy
- vessel integrity and accessibility
- history of previous neck or chest surgery such as mastectomy
- presence of chest trauma
- possible complications.

Veins commonly used as CV insertion sites include the subclavian, internal and external jugular, and brachiocephalic. Rarely are the femoral and brachial veins used. (See *Comparing CV insertion sites*.)

Considering common insertion sites

There are a number of factors the physician will consider when choosing an insertion site for a CV catheter, such as:
- presence of scar tissue
- interference with surgical site or other therapy
- configuration of the lung apices
- patient's lifestyle or daily activities.

In some patients, scar tissue from previous surgery or trauma may prohibit access to major blood vessels or make insertion of a catheter difficult. Or, if the patient is facing surgery in the area of a central vein, another site may need to be chosen. A peripheral site, such as the basilic vein, or a central site on the side of the body unaffected by surgery is a likely alternative.

Another site may be necessary if the patient is receiving other therapy that interferes with the insertion site. For example, if the patient has a tracheostomy, the internal or external jugular site should be avoided because the tracheostomy tapes come too close to these insertion sites. This increases the risk of infection and may cause the catheter to dislodge.

Comparing CV insertion sites

The table below lists the most common insertion sites for a central venous (CV) catheter and the advantages and disadvantages of each.

SITE	ADVANTAGES	DISADVANTAGES
Subclavian vein	• Easy and fast access • Easy to keep dressing in place • High flow rate, which reduces the risk of thrombus	• Close to subclavian artery (If artery is punctured during catheter insertion, hemorrhage can occur.) • Difficulty controlling bleeding • Increased risk of pneumothorax
Internal jugular vein	• Short, direct route to superior vena cava • Catheter stability, resulting in less movement with respiration • Decreased risk of pneumothorax	• Close to the common carotid artery (If artery is punctured during catheter insertion, uncontrolled hemorrhage, emboli, or impedance to flow can result.) • Difficulty keeping the dressing in place • Close to the trachea
External jugular vein	• Easy access, especially in children • Decreased risk of pneumothorax or arterial puncture	• Less direct route • Lower flow rate, which increases the risk of thrombus • Difficulty keeping the dressing in place • Tortuous vein, especially in elderly patients
Cephalic, basilic veins	• Least risk of major complications • Easy to keep the dressing in place	• May be difficult to locate antecubital fossa in obese patients • Difficulty keeping elbow immobile, especially in children

Another site that may be considered is the location of the lung apices. In a patient on mechanical ventilation—especially one receiving positive end-expiratory pressure therapy—intrathoracic pressure increases, which may elevate the lung apices and increase the chance of lung puncture and pneumothorax. A patient with COPD will also have displaced lung apices, and venous access sites outside the thorax should be considered for these patients.

Practical considerations play a role in site selection. For example, a home therapy patient with a PICC may have only one hand with which to work. A woman with a long-term tunneled catheter that exits near her bra straps would have a limited choice of clothing.

Be aware of the catheter's insertion site and the location of the catheter tip so you can be alert for and report potential problems, such as thrombosis, catheter displacement, and infection.

Subclavian vein

The subclavian vein is the most common insertion site for CV therapy. It provides easy access and a short, direct route to the superior vena cava and the CV circulation.

The subclavian vein is a large vein with high-volume blood flow, making clot formation and vessel irritation less likely. The subclavian site also allows the greatest patient mobility after insertion.

When using the subclavian site, the physician inserts the catheter into the vein percutaneously (through the skin and into the vessel with one puncture), threading it into the superior vena cava. This technique requires venipuncture close to the apex of the lung and major vessels of the thorax.

As the catheter enters the skin between the clavicle and first rib, the physician directs the needle toward the angle of Louis, under the clavicle. If the patient moves during insertion, has a chest deformity, or has poor posture, the procedure may be difficult.

Internal jugular vein

The internal jugular vein provides easy access. In many cases, it's the preferred site. This insertion site is commonly used in children but not infants.

The right internal jugular vein provides a more direct route to the superior vena cava than the left internal jugular vein. This site is also used for VAP insertion. However, its proximity to the common carotid artery can lead to serious complications, such as uncontrolled hemorrhage, emboli, or impeded flow, especially if the carotid artery is punctured during catheter insertion (which can cause irreversible brain damage).

Using the internal jugular vein has other drawbacks. For example, it limits the patient's movement and may be a poor choice for home therapy because immobilizing the catheter can be difficult. Because of the location of the internal jugular vein, keeping a dressing in place can also be difficult.

Femoral veins

Femoral veins may be used if other sites aren't suitable. Although the femoral veins are large vessels, using them for catheter insertion entails some complications. Insertion may be difficult, especially in obese patients, and carries the risk of puncturing the local lymph nodes.

Dressing adherence is a big concern when selecting an insertion site. The femoral site inherently carries a greater risk of local infection because of the difficulty of keeping a dressing clean and intact in the groin area.

When a femoral vein is used in CV therapy, the patient's leg needs to be kept straight and movement limited. This prevents bleeding and keeps the catheter from becoming kinked internally or dislodged. Infection can also occur at the insertion site from catheter movement into and out of the incision.

Peripheral veins

The peripheral veins most commonly used as insertion sites include:
- basilic
- cephalic
- external jugular
- median cubital of the antecubital fossa.

Because they're located far from major internal organs and vessels, peripheral veins cause fewer traumatic complications on insertion. However, accessing peripheral veins may cause phlebitis. The tight fit of the catheter in the smaller vessel allows only minimal blood flow around the catheter. Catheter movement may irritate the inner lumen or block it, causing blood pooling (stasis) and thrombus formation.

Although the cephalic vein is more accessible than the basilic vein, the sharp angle makes it more difficult to thread a catheter through. The larger, straighter basilic vein is usually the preferred insertion site. Bedside ultrasound may be used to locate the basilic vein and determine if the vein's condition is appropriate for catheter insertion.

The external jugular vein may provide a CV insertion site. Using the external jugular vein this way presents few complications. However, threading a catheter into the superior vena cava may be difficult because of the sharp angle when entering the subclavian vein from the external jugular vein. For this reason, the catheter tip may remain in the external jugular vein. This position allows high-volume infusions but makes CV pressure measurements less accurate.

Accessing peripheral sites in the antecubital space may limit the patient's mobility because the device exits the skin at the bend of the elbow. Inserting the catheter above the antecubital space allows the patient to be more mobile and prevents kinking but makes it difficult to palpate the veins.

External jugular veins shouldn't be used to administer highly caustic drugs because blood flow around the tip of the catheter may not be strong enough to sufficiently dilute the solutions as they enter the vein.

REINFORCING TEACHING ABOUT CV THERAPY

Ask the patient if he has ever received I.V. therapy before, particularly CV therapy. When describing the procedure to a child, explain it in terms he'll understand. Ask the parents to help with this as well.

If catheter insertion is to take place at the bedside, reinforce the explanation that sterile procedures require the staff to wear gowns, masks, and gloves. Tell your patient he may need to wear a mask as well. If time allows, let your patient, especially a child, try on the mask.

To minimize the patient's anxiety, reinforce how he'll be positioned during the procedure. If the subclavian or jugular vein will be used, he'll be in the Trendelenburg position and a towel may be placed under his back between the scapulae. (In the Trendelenburg position, the head is low and the body and legs are on an inclined surface.) Reassure the patient that he won't be in this position longer than necessary. Stress the position's importance for dilating the veins, which aids insertion and helps prevent insertion-related complications.

Reinforce that the patient should expect a stinging sensation from the local anesthetic and a feeling of pressure during catheter insertion. Explain any other tests that may be done. For example, the physician may obtain a venogram before catheter insertion to check the status of the vessels, especially if the catheter is intended for long-term use. After CV catheter insertion, blood is typically drawn to establish baseline coagulation profiles, and a chest X-ray is done to confirm catheter placement.

If the patient will have the catheter long-term or will be going home with the catheter still inserted, you will need to reinforce patient teaching. A home-therapy coordinator or discharge planner should coordinate teaching and follow-up assessments before and after catheter insertion, but you may need to reinforce the teaching the patient receives about how to care for his catheter himself.

UNDERSTANDING THE EQUIPMENT

Besides the I.V. solution, infusion equipment typically includes an administration set with tubing containing an air-eliminating in-line filter. An infusion pump is used when positive pressure is required, for example, when solutions are given through a CV line at low infusion rates or during intra-arterial infusion.

Some facilities use drip controllers for CV therapy, which permit infusion at a lower pressure. Drip controllers are used most commonly with infants and children, who could suffer serious complications from high-pressure infusion.

If your state nurse practice act and facility policy allow, you may assist with insertion at the patient's bedside, first collect the needed equipment. Most facilities use preassembled disposable trays that include the CV catheter. Although most trays include the necessary equipment, be sure to check. If you don't have a preassembled tray, gather the following items:

- linen-saver pad
- scissors
- povidone-iodine solution
- sterile gauze pads
- chlorhexidine
- local anesthetic
- 3-ml syringe with 25G needle for introduction of anesthetic
- sterile syringe for blood samples
- sterile towels or drapes
- suture material
- sterile dressing
- CV catheter.

Extra syringes and blood sample containers may also be needed if the physician wants to draw venous blood samples during the procedure.

Make sure that everyone participating in the insertion has a mask, a gown, and gloves. You may also need such protection for the patient, especially if there's a risk of site contamination from oral secretions or if the patient can't to cooperate.

Assisting with central venous therapy

Depending on your state nurse practice act and facility policy, you may be permitted to assist with this procedure. Although specific steps may vary, the same basic procedure is used whether catheter insertion is done at the bedside or in the operating room. Before the physician inserts the catheter, you need to position the patient and prepare the insertion site.

Some patients may require sedation for the catheter to be placed. Such patients must be carefully monitored by staff trained in this procedure.

POSITIONING THE PATIENT

The patient is placed in Trendelenburg's position (for insertion in the subclavian or internal jugular veins). This position distends neck and thoracic veins, making them more visible and accessible. Filling the veins also lessens the chance of air emboli because the venous pressure is higher than atmospheric pressure.

If the subclavian vein is to be used, a rolled towel or blanket may be placed between the patient's scapulae. This allows for more direct access and may prevent puncture of the lung apex or adjacent vessels. If a jugular vein is to be used, a rolled blanket may be placed under the patient's opposite shoulder to extend the neck and make anatomic landmarks more visible.

UNDERSTANDING INSERTION SITE PREPARATION

The insertion site is prepared by taking these steps:
- A linen-saver pad is placed under the site to prevent soiling the bed.
- The skin should be free from hair because the follicles can harbor microorganisms.

The intended venipuncture site is prepared with chlorhexidine. A back-and-forth motion is used to prepare the skin. The same area should not be wiped twice, and each gauze pad should be discarded after each complete cycle. The solution should dry completely before the vascular access device insertion proceeds.

After the site is prepared, the physician places sterile drapes around it and, possibly, around the patient's face as well. (This makes the patient's mask unnecessary.) If the patient's face is draped, you can help ease anxiety by uncovering his eyes. The drapes should provide a work area at least as large as the length of the catheter or guide wire.

UNDERSTANDING CATHETER INSERTION

During catheter insertion, if your state nurse practice act or facility policy permits, you may be responsible for monitoring the patient's tolerance of the procedure and providing emotional support. The physician usually prepares the equipment, which comes with a CV access kit and requires sterile technique.

Venous blood samples are drawn after the catheter is inserted. The blood will be placed in the proper sample container or, using a needle or needleless system, a saline lock at the end of the port will be accessed with an evacuated tube. This device draws blood directly into the appropriate tube.

Each time the catheter hub is open to air—such as when the syringe is changed—the patient is told to perform the Valsalva maneuver and the port is clamped to decrease the risk of air embolism. After the catheter is inserted a dressing is applied to the insertion site.

MONITORING THE PATIENT

After the catheter has been inserted, the patient is monitored for complications. Make sure you tailor your data collection to the particular catheter insertion site. For example, if the site is close to major thoracic organs, as with a subclavian or internal jugular site, monitor the patient's respiratory status, watching for dyspnea, shortness of breath, and sudden chest pain.

Catheter insertion can cause arrhythmias if the catheter enters the right ventricle and irritates the heart. For this reason, make sure you monitor the patient's cardiac status. (Arrhythmias usually subside as the catheter is withdrawn.) If the patient isn't attached to a cardiac monitor, palpate the radial artery to detect any rhythm irregularities.

When the end of the catheter rests on the sterile drape, the physician will use one or two sutures to secure the catheter to the skin. Most short-term catheters have preset tabs to hold the sutures. Finally, a chest X-ray is taken to confirm the location of the catheter tip before starting infusions. The line should be capped and flushed with normal saline solution until an X-ray confirms placement. After confirmation, the infusion is begun by connecting the I.V. tubing or intermittent cap to the catheter hub. The flow rate is adjusted as prescribed.

A catheter may be positioned poorly, especially if it's inserted into the internal or external jugular veins. This may cause several problems:
- Dressing changes are more difficult.
- Maintaining an occlusive dressing is impossible.
- The catheter may kink.

UNDERSTANDING CATHETER SITE DRESSING

Sterile technique is maintained during sterile dressing placement over the insertion site of a short-term catheter or exit site of the PICC or tunneled catheter. The dressing is applied using the following steps:

- The site is cleaned with chlorhexidine using the same method as the initial skin preparation.
- The site is covered with a transparent, semipermeable dressing.
- The dressing is sealed with nonporous tape, checking that all edges are well secured.
- The dressing is labeled with the date and time, initials of the person who changed it, and the catheter length.

After the dressing is applied, place the patient in a comfortable position and reassess his status. Elevate the head of the bed 45 degrees to help the patient breathe more easily. Remember to keep the site clean and dry to prevent infection. Remember to keep the dressing occlusive to prevent air embolism and contamination.

UNDERSTANDING INSERTION DOCUMENTATION

All pertinent information is recorded by the RN asssisting the physician in the nurses' notes and on the I.V. flow sheet. What you'll see documented is:

- type of catheter used
- location of insertion
- catheter tip position as confirmed by an X-ray
- patient's tolerance of the procedure
- blood samples taken.

Some facilities recommend documenting the length of catheter remaining outside the body so other nurses can compare the measurements, checking for catheter migration.

Understanding central venous infusion maintenance

Maintaining CV infusions is the RN's responsibility. This includes meticulous care of the CV catheter insertion site as well as of the catheter and tubing.

Maintaining central venous infusions ■ 113

ROUTINE CARE
The following care measures are performed:
- The transparent semipermeable dressing is changed per facility policy or whenever it becomes moist, loose, or soiled.
- The I.V. tubing and solution are changed.
- The catheter is flushed.
- The catheter cap is changed.
- A secondary infusion is administered or blood samples are obtained, if needed.
- Assessment findings and interventions are recorded according to your facility's policy.

Changing dressings
To reduce the risk of infection, gloves and a mask are worn when changing the dressing. The patient and anyone within 9′ (2.7 m) of him should also wear masks. If the patient can't tolerate a facial mask, have him turn his head away from the catheter during the dressing change.

Many facilities use a preassembled dressing-change tray that contains all the needed equipment. If your facility doesn't use this type of tray, the following items are needed:
- chlorhexidine swabs
- transparent semipermeable dressing
- sterile drape
- sterile gloves and masks
- clean gloves
- bag to dispose of removed dressing.

Some CV dressings are changed every 48 hours, but other brands of dressing can remain in place for as long as 7 days, depending on the type of dressing and the facility's policy and procedures. (See *Assisting with a CV dressing change,* pages 114 and 115.)

Changing solutions and tubing
With strict sterile technique maintained, the I.V. solution is changed by the RN every 24 hours and tubing every 72 hours or as directed by your facility's policy. A mask doesn't need to be worn unless there is a contamination risk; for example, if the caregiver has an upper respiratory tract infection.

If possible, the solution and tubing are changed by the RN at the same time. This may not be able to be done if the tubing is damaged or the solution runs out before it's time to change the tubing.

To prevent air embolism, the patient performs the Valsalva maneuver and the port is clamped each time the catheter hub is open

Assisting with a CV dressing change

After the needed equipment is assembled, the step-by-step technique below is followed to safely change a central venous (CV) dressing. If your state nurse practice act or facility policy allows, you may be permitted to assist with this procedure.

GETTING READY
- Hands are washed.
- The patient is placed in a comfortable position.
- A sterile field is prepared, and the bag is opened and placed away from the sterile field but still within reach.

REMOVING THE PREVIOUS
- Clean gloves are used to remove the dressing. The site is inspected for signs of infection. A culture may be taken of any discharge at the site or on the dressing. The dressing and gloves are discarded properly. If an infection is noted, it's reported to the physician immediately and is documented in the nurses' notes.
- The position of the catheter and the insertion site are checked for signs of infiltration or infection, such as redness, swelling, tenderness, or drainage.

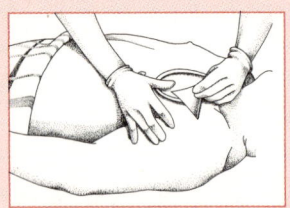

THE PREVIOUS DRESSING IS REMOVED.

---

to air. Many facilities eliminate the need for this by using a connecting tube with a slide clamp between the catheter hub and the I.V. tubing, which allows the I.V. tubing to be clamped during changes.

To change the solution, the following steps are used by the RN:
- A solution container and an alcohol swab are gathered.
- Hands are washed.
- Gloves are put on.
- The cap and seal is removed from the solution container.
- The CV line is clamped.
- The spike is removed quickly from the solution container and reinserted into the new container.
- The new bottle is hung and flow rate adjusted.

APPLYING THE NEW
- Sterile gloves are used to clean the skin around the catheter with chlorhexidine in a back-and-forth or side-to-side motion.
- Solutions containing acetone should not be used because they may cause some catheters to disintegrate.
- If the catheter is taped (not sutured) to the skin, the soiled tape is replaced with sterile tape, using the chevron method. To do so, a strip of tape is cut about ½" (1.3 cm) wide and slid under the catheter, sticky side up. Then the tape is crisscrossed over the top of the catheter. Finally, a second strip of tape is placed over the first strip.
- The site is redressed with a transparent semipermeable dressing.

LABELING
- The dressing is labeled with the date, time, and initials of the person who changed it.
- All used items are discarded properly and the patient is repositioned.

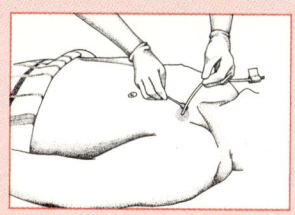

THE INSERTION SITE IS CLEANED.

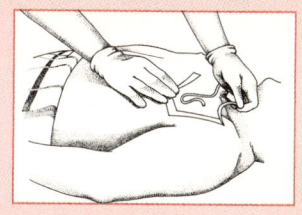

THE SITE IS RE-DRESSED.

To change the tubing, an I.V. administration set, an alcohol wipe, and gloves are gathered. (For information on what is done next, see *Assisting with a CV tubing change,* page 116.)

Flushing the catheter
To maintain patency, the CV catheter must be flushed regularly by the RN with saline solution and according to facility policy. When the system is maintained as an intermittent infusion device, the flushing procedure depends on these variables:
- facility policy
- type of catheter used
- drug administration schedule.

Flushing recommendations vary from every 8 hours to once per day. The recommended amount of flushing solution also varies.

Assisting wtih CV tubing change

After assembling the needed equipment, the following guidelines are used to safely and quickly change central venous (CV) tubing. If your state nurse practice act and facility policy allow, you may assist with this procedure.

- Hands are washed.
- The infusion rate is reduced and the spike from the previous bag is removed. The cover from the new spike is spread loosely over the old spike.
- The old spike is kept in an upright position above the patient's heart and the new spike is inserted into the I.V. container. The system is primed.
- The patient performs the Valsalva maneuver. Quickly, the old tubing is disconnected from the needle or catheter hub, being careful not to dislodge the venipuncture device. If it's difficult to disconnect, a hemostat is used to hold the hub securely while the end of the tubing is twisted and removed. The hemostat should not be clamped shut because the tubing adapter, needle, or catheter hub may crack, which will require a change of equipment and I.V. site.
- The new primed tubing is quickly attached to the venipuncture device using sterile technique.
- The infusion is adjusted to the prescribed rate.
- The new tubing is labeled with the date and time of change.

To change the tubing and solution simultaneously, the following steps are used:
- Hands are washed.
- The new I.V. bag and primed tubing are hung on the I.V. pole.
- The old infusion is stopped.
- The old tubing is quickly disconnected and the new tubing connected, as described above.

Some facilities use a heparinized saline flush solution, available in premixed, 10-ml multidose vials. Recommended concentration strengths vary from 10 units of heparin per milliliter to 1,000 units of heparin per milliliter. The lowest possible effective heparin concentration is used because higher concentrations can interfere with the patient's clotting factors.

Different catheters require not only different amounts of solution but different flushing schedules as well. Generally, a CV catheter with a two-way valve (Groshong tip) is flushed with saline solution once per day when not in use. All lumens of a multilumen catheter (unless it's a valved catheter) must be flushed regularly by the RN with a heparin or saline solution, depending on facility policy and practice. (No flushing is needed with a continuous infusion through a single-lumen catheter.) It's also recommended that a blood return of 3 to 5 ml of free-flowing blood be obtained from the catheter before each use.

Flushing with heparin or normal saline solution should also be performed before and after the administration of incompatible drugs.

Changing caps
CV catheters used for infrequent infusions have intermittent injection caps similar to saline lock adapters used for peripheral I.V. infusion therapy. The frequency of cap changes varies according to facility policy and the number of times that the cap is used. However, the cap should be changed at least every 7 days.

Strict sterile technique is used when changing the cap; repeated puncturing of the injection port increases the risk of infection. Pieces of the rubber stopper may break off after repeated punctures, placing the patient at risk for an embolism. Many needleless caps don't have a rubber port.

Infusing secondary fluids and drawing blood
If other fluids need to be added to the patient's CV infusion, solutions running in the same line need to be compatible and connections must be Luer-locked or well-secured with tape. Secondary I.V. lines may be piggybacked into a side port or Y-port of a primary infusion line instead of being connected directly to the catheter lumen. However, if there is no primary infusion prescribed, the drug may be infused through the CV line. The CV catheter may be used to obtain blood samples, especially if the patient has poor peripheral veins.

Documentation
Assessment findings and interventions are documented according to your facility's policy. (See *Understanding central venous therapy documentation*, page 118.)

PATIENTS REQUIRING ADDITIONAL CARE
Besides routine care measures the following interventions must sometimes be performed by the RN:
- correcting common problems that arise during infusion, such as a damaged or kinked catheter, fluid leaks, and clot formation at the catheter's tip are managed
- meeting the special infusion requirements of home therapy patients, children, and elderly patients
- dealing with potential traumatic complications, such as a pneumothorax and systemic complications such as sepsis. (See *Understanding common problems in CV therapy*, pages 119 and 120.)

> **DOCUMENTATION TIP**
>
> ## Understanding central venous therapy documentation
>
> This type of information is included:
> - the type, amount, and rate of infusion
> - dressing changes, including the appearance and location of the catheter and the site
> - how the patient tolerated the procedure
> - tubing and solution changes
> - cap changes
> - flushing procedures, including any problems encountered and the amount and type of solution used
> - the blood samples collected, including the type and amount.

Common infusion problems

During CV infusions, problems arising from the catheter may require special care measures.

A serrated hemostat will eventually break down silicone rubber and tear the catheter, causing blood to back up and fluid to leak from the device. If air enters the catheter through the tear, an air embolism could result. Catheter tears are prevented by using nonserrated clamps. If the catheter or part of the catheter breaks, cracks, or becomes nonfunctional, the physician may replace the entire CV line with a new one or use a repair kit, if available.

The catheter can become kinked or pinched, either above or beneath the skin. Kinks beneath the skin are detected by X-ray and are usually located between the clavicle and the first rib. The catheter may need to be unsecured and repositioned or replaced.

Never attempt to straighten kinks in stiff catheters such as those made from polyvinyl chloride. These catheters fracture easily. A fractured particle may enter the circulation and act as an embolus. The physician may try to unkink a long-term catheter; this is possible because it's made of pliable silicone rubber. The unkinking is done under guided fluoroscopy using sterile technique.

Catheter kinks may be prevented by taping and positioning the catheter properly. For example, looping the extension tubing once and securing it with tape adjacent to the dressing prevents the catheter from being pulled if the tubing gets entangled. Doing so also helps prevent the catheter from moving or telescoping at the insertion site, a major cause of catheter-related infections and site irritations.

Understanding common problems in CV therapy

Maintaining central venous (CV) therapy requires being prepared to handle potential problems. This table tells how to recognize and manage some problems.

Problem	Possible Causes	Nursing Interventions
Fluid won't infuse	• Closed clamp • Displaced or kinked catheter • Thrombus	• The infusion system and clamps are checked. • The patient's position may be changed. • The patient is instructed to cough, breathe deeply, or perform the Valsalva maneuver. • The dressing is removed and the external portion of the catheter examined. • If a kink isn't apparent, an X-ray order may be obtained. • Blood is withdrawn. • A gentle flush with saline solution is tried. (The physician may order a thrombolytic flush.)
Unable to draw blood	• Closed clamp • Displaced or kinked catheter • Thrombus or fibrin sheath • Catheter movement against vessel wall with negative pressure	• The infusion system and clamps are checked. • The patient's position is changed. • The patient is instructed to cough, breathe deeply, or perform the Valsalva maneuver. • The dressing is removed and the external portion of the catheter examined. • An X-ray order may be obtained to check catheter tip placement.
Fluid leaking at the site	• Displaced or malpositioned catheter • Tear in catheter • Fibrin sheath	• The patient is checked for signs of distress. • The dressing is changed and the site observed for redness. • The physician is notified. • An X-ray order is obtained to check catheter tip placement. • A catheter change may be necessary. • If the tear occurs in a Hickman, Groshong, or Broviac catheter, a repair kit is obtained.

(continued)

Understanding common problems in CV therapy
(continued)

PROBLEM	POSSIBLE CAUSES	NURSING INTERVENTIONS
Disconnected catheter	• Patient moved • Not securely connected to tubing	• A catheter clamp is applied, if available. • A sterile syringe or catheter plug is placed in the catheter hub. • The I.V. extension set is changed. The contaminated tubing is never reconnected. • The catheter hub is cleaned with povidone-iodine or chlorhexidine if the patient has an iodine allergy. The hub shouldn't be soaked. • Clean I.V. tubing or a heparin lock plug is connected to the site. • The infusions are restarted.

If withdrawing blood or infusing fluid is difficult, there may be a clot at the tip of the catheter. This type of sheath impedes the flow of blood and provides a protein-rich environment for bacterial growth.

Occasionally this sheath forms so that fluids infuse easily while blood aspiration is difficult or impossible. The fibrin clot may be dissolved by instilling a thrombolytic. The drug may be instilled by a physician or an RN trained in the procedure.

This procedure is usually recommended for long-term CV catheters because they're difficult and costly to replace, but such an attempt to salvage a device isn't always appropriate or possible.

Pediatric, elderly, and home-care patients

There are a few additional considerations involved in caring for pediatric, elderly, and home-care patients.

Essentially, the same catheters are used in both pediatric and elderly patients. However, these differences are possible:
- catheter length
- lumen size
- insertion sites
- amount of fluid infused.

Maintaining central venous infusions

Long-term CV catheters allow patients to receive fluids, drugs, and blood infusions at home. These catheters have a much longer life because they're less thrombogenic and less prone to infection than short-term devices.

The care procedures used in the home are the same as those used in the hospital, including the use of sterile technique. A candidate for home CV therapy must have:
- a family member or friend who can assist in safe and competent administration of I.V. fluids
- a backup helper
- a suitable home environment
- a telephone
- reliable transportation
- adequate reading skills
- the ability to prepare, handle, store, and dispose of the equipment.

To ensure your patient's safety, patient teaching should begin well before the patient is discharged. After discharge, a home-therapy coordinator provides follow-up care. This helps ensure compliance until the patient or caregiver can independently provide catheter care and infusion therapy at home. Many home-therapy patients learn to care for the catheter themselves and to infuse their own drugs and solutions.

Traumatic and systemic complications

Complications can occur at any time during CV therapy. Traumatic complications such as pneumothorax typically occur on insertion but may not be noticed until after the procedure is completed. Systemic complications such as sepsis typically occur later in therapy. (See *Understanding CV therapy risks* pages 122 to 127.)

Pneumothorax, the most common traumatic complication of catheter insertion, is associated with the insertion of a CV catheter into the subclavian or internal jugular vein. If the patient doesn't have symptoms immediately, pneumothorax is usually discovered on the chest X-ray that confirms catheter placement.

Pneumothorax may be minimal and may not require intervention (unless the patient is on positive-pressure ventilation). A thoracotomy is performed and a chest tube inserted if pneumothorax is large enough to cause these signs and symptoms:
- chest pain
- dyspnea
- cyanosis
- decreased or absent breath sounds on the affected side.

(Text continues on page 124.)

RED FLAG

Understanding CV therapy risks

As with any invasive procedure, central venous (CV) therapy poses risks, including pneumothorax, air embolism, thrombosis, and infection. This table outlines how to recognize, manage, and prevent these complications.

SIGNS AND SYMPTOMS	POSSIBLE CAUSE
PNEUMOTHORAX, HEMOTHORAX, CHYLOTHORAX, OR HYDROTHORAX	
• Chest pain • Dyspnea • Cyanosis • Decreased breath sounds on the affected side • With hemothorax, decreased hemoglobin because of blood pooling • Abnormal chest X-ray	• Lung puncture by catheter during insertion or exchange over a guide wire • Large blood vessel puncture with bleeding inside or outside lung • Lymph node puncture with lymph fluid leakage • Infusion of solution into chest area through perforated catheter
AIR EMBOLISM	
• Respiratory distress • Unequal breath sounds • Weak pulse • Increased central venous pressure (CVP) • Decreased blood pressure • Churning murmur over precordium • Change in or loss of consciousness	• Intake of air into CV system during catheter insertion or tubing changes; inadvertent opening, removal, cutting, or breaking of catheter

Nursing interventions	**Prevention**
• The infusion is stopped and the physician is notified. • The catheter is removed. • Oxygen is administered. • Assist the physician with chest tube insertion • Interventions are documented.	• The patient should be positioned head down with a towel roll between scapulae to dilate and expose the internal jugular or subclavian vein as much as possible during catheter insertion. • Early signs of fluid infiltration, such as swelling in the shoulder, neck, chest, and arm area should be assessed. • The patient should be immobilized with adequate preparation for procedure and restraint during procedure; active patients may need to be sedated or taken to the operating room for CV catheter insertion. • CV catheter position should be confirmed by X-ray.
• The catheter is clamped immediately. • The catheter exit site is covered. • The patient is turned on his left side, head down, so that air can enter the right atrium, preventing it from entering the pulmonary artery. • The patient shouldn't perform Valsalva's maneuver. (Large intake of air worsens the situation.) • Oxygen is administered. • The physician is notified. • Interventions are documented.	• Air should be purged from tubing before hookup. • The patient should be taught to perform Valsalva's maneuver during catheter insertion and tubing changes (bear down or strain and hold breath to increase CVP). • Air-eliminating filters should be used proximal to the patient. • An infusion-control device should be used with air detection capability. • Luer-lock tubing and tape connections or locking devices should be used for all connections.

(continued)

Understanding CV therapy risks *(continued)*

SIGNS AND SYMPTOMS

POSSIBLE CAUSE

THROMBOSIS

- Edema at puncture site
- Ipsilateral swelling of arm, neck, and face
- Pain
- Fever, malaise
- Tachycardia

- Sluggish flow rate
- Hematopoietic status of patient
- Preexisting limb edema
- Infusion of irritating solutions
- Irritation of tunica intima
- Repeated use of same vein or long-term use
- Preexisting cardiovascular disease (such as atrial fibrillation)
- Vein irritation during insertion

LOCAL INFECTION

- Redness, warmth, tenderness, and swelling at insertion or exit site
- Possible exudate of purulent material
- Local rash or pustules
- Fever, chills, malaise

- Failure to maintain sterile technique during catheter insertion or care
- Failure to comply with dressing change protocol
- Wet or soiled dressing remaining on site
- Immunosuppression
- Irritated suture line

Initially, the patient may be asymptomatic; signs of distress gradually show up as pneumothorax gets larger. For this reason the patient should be closely monitored with his breath sounds auscultated for at least 8 hours after catheter insertion.

If unchecked, pneumothorax may progress to tension pneumothorax, a medical emergency. The patient may exhibit these signs:

Nursing interventions	**Prevention**
● The physician is notified. (He may remove the catheter.) ● A thrombolytic may be infused to dissolve the clot. ● Thrombosis is verified with diagnostic studies. ● The limb on the affected side is not used for subsequent venipuncture. ● Interventions are documented.	● Flow should be maintained through the catheter at a steady rate with an infusion pump or should be flushed at regular intervals. ● It should be verified that the catheter tip is in superior vena cava before using the catheter.
● Temperature is monitored frequently. ● The site is cultured. ● The site is re-dressed aseptically. ● Possibly, an antibiotic ointment is applied locally. ● Systemic treatment with antibiotics or antifungals, depending on the culture results and the physician's orders. ● The catheter may be removed. ● Interventions are documented.	● Strict aseptic technique should be maintained. Gloves, masks, and gowns are used when appropriate. ● Dressing change protocols should be adhered to. ● The patient should be taught about restrictions on swimming, bathing, and so on. (Patients with adequate white blood cell counts can do these activities if the physician allows.) ● Wet or soiled dressings should be changed immediately. ● The dressing should be changed more frequently if the catheter is located in the femoral area or near a tracheostomy. ● Tracheostomy care should be completed after catheter care.

(continued)

- acute respiratory distress
- asymmetrical chest wall movement
- a tracheal shift away from the affected side.

A chest tube must be inserted immediately before respiratory and cardiac decompensation occurs.

The second most common life-threatening complication is arterial puncture. Arterial puncture may lead to hemothorax and inter-

> **Understanding CV therapy risks** *(continued)*
>
> | SIGNS AND SYMPTOMS | POSSIBLE CAUSE |
> | --- | --- |
> | **SYSTEMIC INFECTION** | |
> | • Fever, chills without other apparent reason
• Leukocytosis
• Nausea, vomiting
• Malaise
• Elevated urine glucose level | • Contaminated catheter or infusate
• Failure to maintain sterile technique during solution hook
• Frequent opening of catheter or long-term use of single l access
• Immunosuppression |

nal bleeding; these problems may not be detected immediately. Hemothorax is treated like pneumothorax except that the chest tube is inserted lower in the chest to help evacuate the blood.

Left untreated, internal bleeding from arterial puncture leads to hypovolemic shock. Signs and symptoms include:
- increased heart rate
- decreased blood pressure
- cool, clammy skin
- obvious swelling in the neck or chest
- mental confusion (especially if the common carotid arteries are involved)
- hematoma, which puts pressure on the trachea and adjacent vessels.

There are a few additional, but rare, complications of CV therapy:
- tracheal puncture from insertion of a catheter into the subclavian vein
- fistula between the innominate vein and the subclavian artery from perforation by the guide wire on insertion into the vessel

Nursing interventions	**Prevention**
● Central and peripheral blood cultures are drawn; if cultures match, the catheter is primary source of sepsis and should be removed. ● If cultures don't match but are positive, the catheter may be removed or the infection may be treated through the catheter. ● The patient is treated with antibiotic regimen, as ordered. ● The tip of the catheter is cultured, if removed. ● Other sources of infection are assessed. ● Vital signs are closely monitored. ● Interventions are documented.	● Infusate should be examined for cloudiness and turbidity before infusing. ● The fluid container should be checked for leaks. ● Urine glucose level should be monitored in a patient receiving total parenteral nutrition; if greater than 2+, early sepsis should be suspected. ● Strict aseptic technique should be used for hookup and disconnection of fluids. ● The catheter may be changed frequently to decrease the chance of infection. ● The system should be kept closed as much as possible. ● The patient should be taught aseptic technique.

- chylothorax from a punctured lymph node causing lymph fluid to leak into the pleural cavity
- hydrothorax (or infusion of solution into the chest)
- thrombosis
- local infection.

Catheter-related sepsis is the most serious systemic complication, having these outcomes:

- septic shock
- multisystem organ failure
- death.

Most sepsis attributed to CV catheters is caused by skin surface organisms, such as *Staphylococcus epidermidis, S. aureus,* and *Candida albicans.*

Strict sterile technique and close observation are the best ways to prevent sepsis. The catheter insertion site should be checked regularly for signs of localized infection, such as redness, drainage, or tenderness along the catheter path. If the patient shows signs of generalized infection such as unexplained fever, blood cultures should be drawn from a peripheral site as well as from the device itself, according to your facility's policy.

If catheter-related sepsis is suspected, the catheter may be removed and a new one inserted in a different site. The catheter tip is cultured after removal. Antibiotics are given and blood is drawn for repeat cultures after the antibiotic course is complete.

PICC-specific complications

PICC therapy causes fewer and less severe complications than other CV lines. Pneumothorax is extremely rare because the insertion site is peripheral. Catheter-related sepsis is usually related to site contamination.

Mechanical phlebitis — painful inflammation of a vein — may be the most common PICC complication. It usually occurs during the first 72 hours after PICC insertion and is more common in left-sided insertions and when a large-gauge catheter is used.

If the patient develops mechanical phlebitis, apply warm moist compresses to his upper arm, elevate the extremity, and restrict activity to mild exercise. If the phlebitis continues or worsens, the catheter must be removed.

Bacterial phlebitis can occur with PICCs, but this usually occurs later in the infusion therapy. If drainage occurs at the insertion site and the patient's temperature increases, notify the physician. The catheter may have to be removed.

Expect minimal bleeding from the PICC insertion site for the first 24 hours. Persistent bleeding needs additional evaluation. Notify the prescriber if bleeding persists. A pressure dressing should be left in place over the insertion site for at least 24 hours. If the bleeding stops after that, the dressing can be changed and a new transparent dressing applied without a gauze pressure dressing.

Some patients complain of pain at the PICC insertion site, usually because the device is located in an area of frequent flexion. Pain may be treated by applying warm compresses and restricting activities until the patient becomes adjusted to the presence of the PICC.

Air embolism in PICC therapy is less common than in traditional CV lines because the line is inserted below heart level.

STOPPING CENTRAL VENOUS THERAPY

A physician or an RN may remove the catheter, and depending on your state's nurse practice act, your facility's policy, and the type of catheter, you may assist wtih the procedure. Long-term catheters and implanted devices are always removed by a physician, but PICC lines may be removed by a qualified nurse.

For an order to stop continuous infusion therapy and begin intermittent infusion therapy, the same procedure as for peripheral I.V. therapy is used. An intermittent infusion device is used to convert the line from continuous to intermittent therapy.

Removing the catheter

Catheter removal starts with a couple of precautions. First, as directed by facility policy, the patient's record or other documentation (such as the nurses' notes, physicians' notes, or the written X-ray report) is checked for the most recent placement confirmed by an X-ray to trace the catheter's path as it exits the body. If a complication such as uncontrolled bleeding occurs during catheter removal, backup supplies and assistance are made available. This complication is common in patients with coagulopathies. Before the catheter is removed, the procedure is explained to the patient. He'll need to turn his face away from the site and perform the Valsalva maneuver when the catheter is withdrawn.

Before removing the catheter, the necessary equipment is gathered, including:
- sterile gauze
- clean gloves
- sterile gloves
- forceps
- sterile scissors
- povidone-iodine solution
- alcohol swabs
- transparent, semipermeable dressing
- tape.

If the tip of the catheter was swabed and sent for culture, a sterile specimen container is also needed. (See *Understanding CV catheter removal,* page 130.)

After removing the catheter, the following should be documented:
- patient tolerance
- condition of the catheter, including the length
- time of discontinuation of therapy
- cultures ordered and sent
- any complications that occurred, symptoms of infection, or other pertinent information.

Understanding CV catheter removal

After equipment is assembled, the following step-by-step guidelines are used to safely remove a central venous (CV) catheter.

GETTING READY
- The patient is placed in a supine position to prevent emboli.
- Hands are washed and clean gloves are put on.
- All infusions are turned off.
- The old dressing is removed.
- The site is inspected for signs of drainage or inflammation.

REMOVING THE CATHETER
- The sutures are clipped and the catheter is removed in a slow, even motion. The patient performs Valsalva's maneuver as the catheter is withdrawn to prevent air emboli.
- Povidone-iodine or antibiotic ointment is applied to the insertion site to seal it.
- The catheter is inspected to see if any pieces broke off during the removal. If so, the physician is notified immediately and the patient monitored closely for signs of distress. If a culture is to be obtained, the distal end of the catheter is swabbed with a sterile swab and sent to the laboratory for culture.
- A transparent semipermeable dressing is placed over the site. The dressing is labeled with the date and time of the removal and the initials of the person who removed the catheter.
- The used I.V. tubing and equipment are disposed of properly.

MONITORING THE PATIENT
Insidious bleeding may develop after the catheter is removed. Remember that some vessels, such as the subclavian vein, aren't easily compressed. Within 72 hours, the site should be sealed and the risk of air emboli should be past; however, a dry dressing may still need to be applied to the site.

A notation on the nursing care plan to recheck the patient and insertion site frequently for the next few hours should be made. The patient should be checked for signs of respiratory decompensation, possibly indicating air emboli, and for signs of bleeding, such as blood on the dressing, decreased blood pressure, increased heart rate, paleness, or diaphoresis.

NOTEWORTHY
The time and date of the catheter removal and any complications that occurred, such as catheter shearing, bleeding, or respiratory distress should be documented. The length of the catheter and signs of blood, drainage, redness, or swelling at the site, should also be recorded.

VAP implantation and infusion

Implanted under the skin, a VAP consists of a silicone catheter attached to a reservoir, covered by a self-sealing silicone rubber septum. Implanting a VAP requires surgery. The device may be placed in the arm, chest, abdomen, flank of the chest, or thigh.

Usually, a VAP is used to deliver these intermittent infusions:
- chemotherapy
- I.V. fluids
- pain control
- drugs
- blood products.

VAPs may also be used to deliver TPN. When giving TPN, the access site needs to be closely monitored to assess skin integrity. VAPs may also be used for long-term antibiotic therapy or to obtain blood samples.

To reduce the number of punctures to a VAP, an intermittent infusion device or lock may be used. VAPs should be used cautiously in patients with a high risk of developing an allergic reaction or infection.

SELECTING THE EQUIPMENT

The VAP selected for a patient depends on these two variables:
- the type of therapy needed
- how often the port needs to be accessed. (Typically, VAPs are used for intermittent infusions and only require access during the prescribed therapy.)

The selection of infusion equipment depends partly on the type of VAP selected and the implantation site. Generally, the same infusion equipment as in peripheral I.V. and CV therapy is used, including an infusion solution and an administration set with tubing.

Depending on the patient's size and the type of therapy, a VAP catheter with one or two large or small lumens may be chosen. VAPs come in two basic types: top entry and side entry.

In a top-entry VAP (such as the Med-I-Port, Port-A-Cath, Passport, and Infuse-A-Port), the needle is inserted perpendicular to the reservoir. In a side-entry VAP (such as the S.E.A. Port), the needle is inserted almost parallel to the reservoir. Top-entry VAPs are more commonly used. (See *A close look at a top-entry VAP,* page 132.)

The VAP reservoir may be made of:
- titanium (Port-A-Cath)
- stainless steel (Q-Port)
- molded plastic (Infuse-A-Port).

A close look at a top-entry VAP

In a top-entry vascular access port (VAP), the most commonly used port type, the needle is inserted perpendicular to the reservoir.

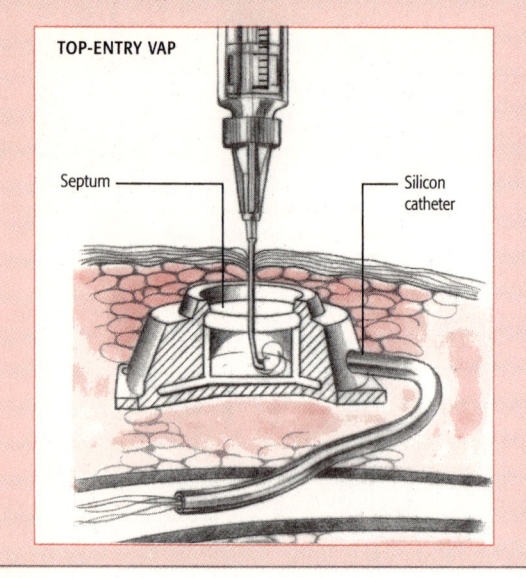

TOP-ENTRY VAP

Septum

Silicon catheter

The type of VAP reservoir used depends on the patient's therapeutic needs. For example, a patient undergoing magnetic resonance imaging should have a device made of titanium or plastic, instead of stainless steel, to avoid distorting test results.

To avoid damaging the port's silicone rubber septum, only noncoring needles are used. A noncoring needle has an angled or deflected point that slices the septum on entry, rather than coring it as a conventional needle does. When the noncoring needle is removed, the septum reseals itself. (See *A close look at noncoring needles*.)

Noncoring needles come with metal or plastic hubs in straight or right-angle configurations, with or without an extension set. Each configuration comes in various lengths (depending on the depth of septum implantation) and gauges (depending on the rate of infusion). (See *Choosing the right VAP needle*, page 134.)

A close look at noncoring needles

Unlike a conventional hypodermic needle, a noncoring needle has a deflected point, which slices the port's septum instead of coring it. Noncoring needles come in two types: straight and right angle.

Generally, you can expect a right-angle needle to be used with a top-entry port and a straight needle with a side-entry port. When administering a bolus injection or continuous infusion, an extension set will also be used.

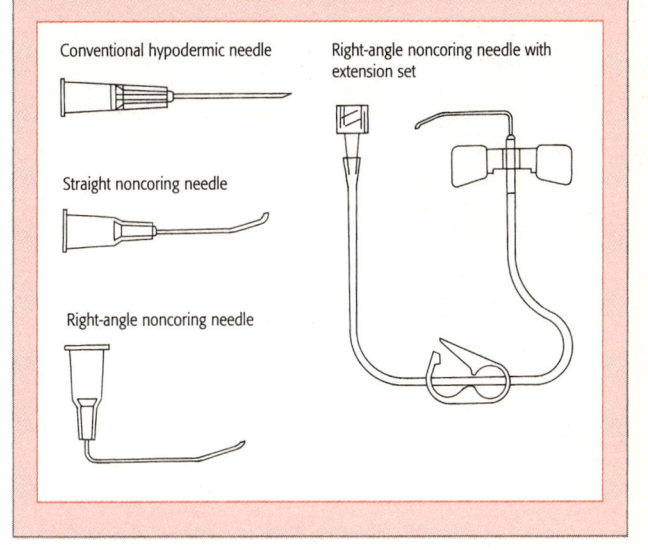

Conventional hypodermic needle

Straight noncoring needle

Right-angle noncoring needle

Right-angle noncoring needle with extension set

An over-the-needle catheter allows continuous access to the port. This style of catheter is more comfortable for the patient and there's less risk of the device migrating out of the septum.

In an over-the-needle catheter, a solid-spike introducer and flexible catheter are passed through the silicone septum. Then the introducer is removed and the flexible catheter is positioned along the contour of the patient's chest wall.

VAP IMPLANTATION

A physician surgically implants the VAP, usually using local anesthesia with conscious sedation. Occasionally, general anesthesia is used.

When implanting the VAP, the physician will perform the following steps:

Choosing the right VAP needle

When choosing a vascular access port (VAP) needle, experts recommend:
- 19G needles for blood infusion or withdrawal
- 20G needles for most infusions (other than blood infusion or withdrawal), including total parenteral nutrition
- 22G needles for flushing.

Remember that you should use only noncoring needles with a VAP.

RIGHT ANGLE VS. STRAIGHT
A right-angle noncoring needle is most commonly used; rarely, a longer needle, such as a straight 2" noncoring needle, is used to access a deeply implanted port.

Either a straight needle or a right-angle needle to inject a bolus into a top-entry port can be used. For continuous infusions, however, experts recommend using a right-angle needle because it's easily secured to the patient. Side-entry ports are designed for use with straight noncoring needles only.

- Make a small incision and introduce the catheter into the superior vena cava through either the subclavian, jugular, or cephalic vein. Fluoroscopy is used to verify placement of the catheter tip.
- Create a subcutaneous pocket over a bony prominence on the chest wall and tunnel the catheter to the pocket.
- Connect the catheter to the reservoir, place the reservoir in the pocket, and flush it with heparinized saline solution.
- Suture the reservoir to the underlying fascia and close the incision.

A dressing is then applied to the wound site, according to your facility's policy and procedures. Once the implantation site is healed, routine dressing practices are used when the VAP is in use.

Preparing the patient

Because VAP implantation is an operating-room procedure, patient teaching should cover preoperative and postoperative instructions. Use the following pointers to reinforce teaching before VAP implantation:

- Make sure the patient understands the procedure, its benefits, and what is expected of him after the implantation. Answer questions and give additional information about teaching the physician has already given. You'll also need to soothe the patient's fears and answer questions about movement restrictions, cosmet-

ic concerns, and maintenance regimens. Clear explanations help ensure the patient's cooperation.
- Explain to the patient the purpose of a venogram, which may be ordered to determine the best vessel to use. The venogram is performed while the patient is under anesthesia and before postoperative swelling occurs, allowing immediate use of the device.
- Make sure you describe how the patient will be positioned during the procedure.

Obtaining consent

Most facilities require a signed informed consent form before any invasive procedure. Tell the patient he'll be asked to sign a consent form and explain what this means.

The physician obtains consent. Before the patient signs, make sure he understands the procedure. If not, delay signing until you or the physician clarifies the procedure and the patient demonstrates understanding.

Rarely, a patient requires emergency VAP implantation. The consent form can be signed by the next of kin or legal guardian. In this case, your teaching may be deferred until after the device is in place.

Reinforce prior teaching of the following postoperative care topics:
- Remind the patient that once the device is in place, he'll have to keep scheduled appointments to have the port heparinized. Another option is to teach him or his family how to heparinize the port.
- Tell the patient to report signs and symptoms of systemic infection, such as fever, malaise, and flulike symptoms, and of local infection, such as redness, tenderness, and drainage at the port or tunnel track site.
- The patient will need to receive prophylactic antibiotics before undergoing any dental or surgical procedures to prevent contamination and colonization of the VAP. Tell him to inform his dentist or physician that he has an implanted device. Tell the patient to carry identification material pertaining to specific care protocols, serial number, and model of the VAP.
- Teach the patient to recognize and report signs and symptoms of infiltration, such as pain or swelling at the site, especially if he'll be receiving continuous infusions. Stress the need for immediate intervention to avoid damaging the tissue surrounding the port, especially if the patient is receiving vesicant drugs.

Monitoring the patient

After the VAP is implanted, observe the patient for several hours. The device can be used immediately after placement. Some swelling and tenderness may persist for about 72 hours, making the device initially difficult to palpate and slightly uncomfortable for the patient.

The incision requires routine postoperative care for 7 to 10 days. Assess the implantation site for these signs:
- infection
- clotting
- redness
- device rotation
- skin irritation.

VAP INFUSION

To give an infusion with a VAP, first the physician accesses the port with the appropriate needle in the operating room. When infusion therapy is started, equipment will be set up and the site will be prepared.

Preparing the equipment

If your state nurse practice act and facility policy allows you to set up infusion equipment, these steps are followed:
- The tubing is attached to the solution container.
- The tubing is primed with fluid.
- If setting up an intermittent system, two syringes are filled: one with 5 ml of normal saline solution and the other with 5 ml of 100 units/ml heparin solution.
- The noncoring needle and extension set are primed with the saline solution from the syringe. (The tubing is primed and purged of air using strict sterile technique.)
- After the tubing is primed, all the connections are rechecked for tightness. Make sure all open ends are covered with sealed caps.

Preparing the site

To prepare the insertion site, obtain an implantable port access kit, if your facility uses them. If a kit isn't available, gather the necessary equipment:
- sterile gloves
- three alcohol swabs
- three povidone-iodine swabs
- sterile 3" × 3" gauze pad
- sterile 1" × 1" gauze pad

VAP implantation and infusion

- transparent dressing
- tape
- mask
- sterile drape.

When the access site is ready to prepare, the following precautions are taken:

- A sterile field for the sterile supplies is established and the area around the port is inspected for signs of infection or skin breakdown.
- An ice pack may be placed over the area for several minutes to numb the site.
- A thick layer of the anesthetic cream is applied over the injection port and covered with a transparent dressing. This cream is removed completely before putting on sterile gloves and preparing the access site.

To prepare the access site, these steps are followed:

- Hands are washed thoroughly and sterile gloves are applied.
- The area is cleaned with an alcohol swab, starting at the center of the port and working outward with a firm back-and forth, or swiping, motion. Repeat this procedure twice more, allowing the alcohol to dry thoroughly.
- Clean the area with a povidone-iodine swab in the same manner described above. This procedure is done twice. Most importantly, the povidone-iodine is allowed to dry.
- If facility policy calls for a local anesthetic, the patient's record is checked for possible allergies. If indicated, the insertion site is anesthetized by injecting 0.1 ml of lidocaine (Xylocaine), without epinephrine, intradermally. Transdermal analgesia may also be used but must be applied about an hour before the access procedure.

Accessing the site

If your state nurse practice act and facility policy allows you to access a top-entry VAP, a right-angle noncoring needle and a 5-ml syringe filled with saline solution are used. (See *How a top-entry VAP is accessed,* page 138.)

The same procedure is used to gain access to a side-entry port. However, the needle is inserted parallel to the reservoir instead of perpendicular to it.

While the patient is hospitalized, an intermittent infusion cap or lock may be attached to the end of the extension set. The cap contains a clamping mechanism to provide ready access for intermittent infusions.

> **BEST PRACTICE**
>
> ## How a top-entry VAP is accessed
>
> Check your state nurse practice act and facility policy to see if you are permitted to perform this procedure. After assembling equipment, the following step-by-step guidelines are followed to safely and securely access a top-entry vascular access port (VAP):
>
> - The area over the port is palpated to locate the septum. Optimally, the patient should be sitting up with his back supported.
> - The port is anchored between the thumb and the first two fingers of the nondominant hand. Then, using the dominant hand, the needle is aimed at the center of the device in between thumb and first finger.
> - The needle is inserted perpendicular to the port septum, as shown. The needle is pushed through the skin and septum until it reaches the bottom of the reservoir. The metal back of the port will be felt.
> - The needle placement is checked by aspirating for a blood return.
> - If blood can't be obtained, the needle is removed and the procedure repeated. Inability to obtain blood might indicate that the catheter is malfunctioning. If blood can't be obtained, the physician is notified: A fibrin sheath on the distal end of the catheter may be blocking the opening.
> - The device is flushed with normal saline solution. If swelling is detected or if the patient reports pain at the site, the needle is removed and the physician notified.

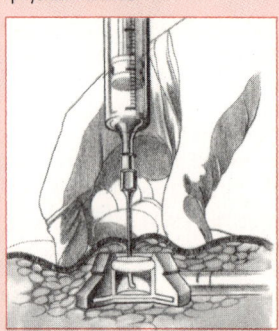

In addition to saving valuable nursing time, an accessed VAP reduces the discomfort of reaccessing the port. It also prolongs the life of the port septum by decreasing the number of needle punctures.

Giving a bolus injection

To give a bolus injection, first check your state nurse practice act and facility policy, then, the following is needed:
- 10-ml syringe filled with saline solution
- syringe containing the prescribed medication
- syringe filled with the appropriate heparin flush solution (if indicated). (See *How a bolus injection is administered by VAP*.)

How a bolus injection is administered by VAP

The step-by-step instructions below show how a bolus injection via a vascular access port (VAP) is given safely and accurately.

- A 10-ml syringe filled with saline solution is attached to the end of the extension set and all the air is removed. The extension set is attached to a noncoring needle.
- Blood return is checked and then the port is flushed with saline solution, according to your facility's policy. (Some facilities require flushing the port with heparin solution first.) If no blood is obtained, the physician is notified.
- The extension set is clamped and the saline solution syringe removed.
- The medication syringe is connected to the extension set. The clamp is opened and the drug injected, as ordered.

EXAMINE, CLAMP, AND FLUSH
- The skin surrounding the needle is examined for signs of infiltration, such as swelling or tenderness. If these signs are noted, the injection is stopped and appropriate intervention is performed.
- When the injection is complete, the extension set is clamped and the medication syringe is removed.
- The clamp is opened and flushed with 5 ml of saline solution after each drug injection to minimize drug incompatibility reactions.
- As your facility policy directs, the port is flushed with heparin solution.

WRITE IT DOWN
The injection is documented according to your facility's policy and includes the following information: the type and amount of medication injected, the time of the injection, the appearance of the site, the patient's tolerance of the procedure, and any pertinent nursing interventions.

Starting continuous infusion

To prepare for a continuous infusion with a VAP, gather the necessary equipment, including:
- prescribed I.V. solution or drug
- I.V. administration set with an air-eliminating filter, if ordered
- 10-ml syringe filled with saline solution
- antibacterial ointment (such as povidone-iodine ointment), if ordered
- adhesive tape
- sterile 2" × 2" gauze pad
- sterile tape or adhesive skin closures
- transparent semipermeable dressing.

The access needle should be attached with an extension set that has a clamp. (See *How a continuous VAP infusion is administered.*)

MAINTAINING VAP INFUSIONS

If your state nurse practice act and facility policy allows you to maintain infusion therapy with a VAP, the following care measures are performed:
- The VAP is flushed with heparin solution if the VAP is used intermittently.
- The site is assessed at established intervals.
- The dressing is changed per the facility's policy or whenever the dressing's integrity is compromised.
- Common equipment problems and patient complications are managed.
- Therapy is stopped when ordered, or the VAP is converted to an intermittent system to keep the device patent until it's needed again.

Flushing a VAP

These guidelines are used to determine when to flush a VAP:
- If your patient is receiving a continuous or prolonged infusion, the port is flushed after infusions and the dressing and needle or needleless device is changed every 7 days. The tubing and solution are changed according to your facility's policy.
- If your patient is receiving an intermittent infusion, the port is flushed periodically with saline and heparin solutions. Keep in mind that the Groshong-type VAP doesn't require heparinization.
- To help prevent clot formation in the device, the VAP is flushed with heparin solution after each saline solution flush. When the VAP isn't accessed, it's flushed once every 4 weeks.

To flush the VAP, the necessary equipment is gathered:
- 22G noncoring needle with an extension set
- 10-ml syringe filled with 5 ml of sterile normal saline solution
- 10-ml syringe filled with 5 ml of heparin flush solution (100 units/ml).

Each syringe should be carefully labeled so they aren't confused.

The injection site is prepared, as described above. Then these steps are followed:
- The 10-ml syringe with 5 ml of normal saline solution is attached to the extension set and noncoring needle, applying gentle pressure to the plunger to expel all air from the set.
- The area over the port is palpated to locate it and the port is accessed.

How a continuous VAP infusion is administered

The step-by-step instructions below show how to administer a continuous vascular access port (VAP) infusion safely and accurately.

ASSEMBLE, REMOVE, FLUSH, CONNECT, AND BEGIN
- The equipment is assembled.
- The air is removed from the extension set by priming it with an attached syringe of saline solution. Then the extension set is attached to a noncoring needle.
- The port system is flushed with saline solution. The extension set is clamped and the syringe removed.
- The administration set is connected and the connections are secured with tape, if necessary.
- The extension set is unclamped and the infusion begun.

ADJUST AND EXAMINE
- A gauze pad is placed under the needle hub if it doesn't lie flush with the skin, as shown below left.
- To help prevent needle dislodgment, the needle is secured to the skin with sterile tape or adhesive skin closures, as shown below right.
- A transparent semipermeable dressing is applied over the needle insertion site.

- The site is examined carefully for infiltration. If the patient complains of burning, stinging, or pain at the site, the infusion is discontinued and appropriate intervention performed.

OBTAIN, CLAMP, AND ATTACH
- When the solution container is empty, a new I.V. solution container is obtained, as ordered, with primed I.V. tubing.
- The extension set is clamped and the old I.V. tubing is removed.
- The new I.V. tubing is attached to the solution container and the extension set. The clamps are opened and the infusion rate adjusted.

WRITE IT DOWN
The infusion is documented according to your facility's policy, including the following information: the type, amount, rate, and time of infusion; the patient's tolerance of the procedure; the appearance of the site; and any pertinent nursing interventions.

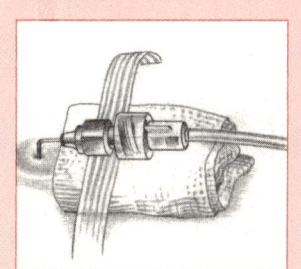

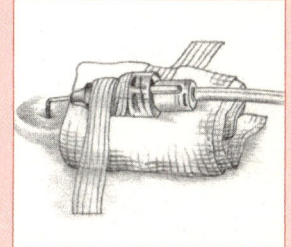

> ### Thrombolytics may be forbidden
>
> Because thrombolytics increase the risk of bleeding, they may be contraindicated in patients who have had surgery within the past 10 days; who have active internal bleeding, such as GI bleeding; or who have experienced central nervous system damage, such as infarction, hemorrhage, trauma, surgery, or primary or metastatic disease within the past 2 months.

- After aspirating for blood return the VAP is first flushed with normal saline solution to confirm patency, then flushed with the heparin solution.
- While stabilizing the VAP with two fingers, the noncoring needle is withdrawn.

Obtaining blood samples
Blood samples can be obtained from an implanted VAP with either a syringe or an evacuated tube.

Clearing the VAP
If clotting threatens to block the VAP, making flushing and infusions sluggish, the physician may order a thrombolytic to clear the port and catheter. if your state nurse practice act and facility policy allows you to assist with this procedure, gather the following:

To clear the VAP, this equipment is needed:
- a 20G or 22G noncoring needle with an extension set
- a syringe filled with a thrombolytic
- an empty 10-ml syringe
- a 5-ml syringe and 10-ml syringe, both filled with saline solution
- a sterile syringe filled with heparin flush solution.

These steps are followed by the physician or RN to clear the port and catheter:
- The area over the port is palpated and the VAP is accessed.
- Blood return is checked.
- The VAP is flushed with 5 ml of saline solution, and the extension tubing is clamped.
- The syringe containing the thrombolytic is attached and the extension tubing is unclamped.
- The thrombolytic solution is instilled using a gentle pull-push motion on the syringe plunger to mix the solution in the access equipment, VAP, and catheter.
- The extension set is clamped and the solution is left in place for 15 minutes (may be up to 30 minutes in some facilities).

> **DOCUMENTATION TIP**
> ### Documenting vascular access port infusions
>
> Assessment findings and interventions are documented according to your facility's policy. The following information is included:
> - type, amount, rate, and duration of the infusion
> - appearance of the site
> - problems and the steps taken to resolve them
> - needle gauge and length and dressing changes for continuous infusions
> - type and amount of blood samples obtained
> - patient-teaching topics covered and the patient's response to the procedure.

- Then an empty 10-ml syringe is attached, the extension set is unclamped, and the thrombolytic and clot are aspirated with the 10-ml syringe. This syringe is discarded to prevent the accidental injection of the thrombolytic into the systemic circulation.
- If the clot can't be aspirated, the procedure is tried again in 15 minutes. If the patient's platelet count is greater than 20,000/ml, a thrombolytic solution can be safely instilled as many as three times in a 4-hour period. If the patient's platelet count is less than 20,000/ml, the procedure is repeated only once in a 4-hour period.
- After the blockage is cleared, the catheter is flushed with at least 10 ml of saline solution and then flushed with heparin solution.

A thrombolytic is contraindicated in patients with these conditions:
- active bleeding
- intracranial neoplasms
- hypersensitivity to thrombolytics
- liver disease
- subacute bacterial endocarditis or visceral tumors
- stroke in the past 2 months. (See *Thrombolytics may be forbidden*.)

Assessment findings and interventions are documented according to your facility's policy. (See *Documenting vascular access port infusions*.)

PREVENTING PROBLEMS

Routine care measures are subject to a few glitches. Commonly, problems may arise during an infusion with a VAP that won't allow the following events to occur:
- flush the VAP

- withdraw blood from the VAP
- palpate and access the VAP. (See *Understanding common VAP problems.*)

Generally, the procedures for implanting and maintaining a VAP are the same for pediatric and elderly patients as for adult patients, with one big exception: For children, general anesthesia may be used during implantation.

A home-care patient requires thorough teaching about procedures and follow-up visits from a home-care nurse to ensure compliance, safety, and successful treatment.

If the patient will access the port himself, explain that the most uncomfortable part of the procedure is inserting the needle into the skin. Once the needle has penetrated the skin, the patient will feel some pressure but little pain. Eventually, the skin over the port becomes desensitized from frequent needle punctures. Until then, the patient may want to use a topical anesthetic.

Stress the importance of pushing the needle into the port until the needle bevel touches the back of the port. Many patients tend to stop short of the back of the port, leaving the needle bevel in the rubber septum. This can cause blockage or can slow the infusion rate.

A patient with a VAP faces risks similar to those of a traditional CV catheter, such as infection and infiltration. Teach the patient or caregiver how to recognize signs and symptoms of these complications. Make sure that they know how to intervene or how to contact the home health agency. (See *Understanding complications of VAP therapy,* pages 146 and 147.)

INTERRUPTING VAP THERAPY

If your state nurse practice act and facility policy allows you to interrupt VAP therapy the access needle is removed from a VAP only after it has been flushed for maintenance. Although there is usually little or no bloody drainage when the access needle is removed, these precautions are observed:
- Gloves are worn.
- The needle is disposed of properly.
- A small dressing is placed temporarily over the VAP site.

Stopping a VAP

To prepare to stop therapy, this necessary equipment is gathered:
- 10-ml syringe filled with 5 ml of normal saline solution
- 10-ml syringe filled with 5 ml of sterile 100 units/ml heparin flush solution
- sterile gloves

Understanding common VAP problems

To maintain a vascular access port (VAP), common problems must be handled. This table outlines problems you may encounter, their possible causes, and the appropriate nursing interventions.

PROBLEM AND POSSIBLE CAUSES	NURSING INTERVENTIONS
INABILITY TO FLUSH OR WITHDRAW BLOOD	
• Kinked tubing or closed clamp	• The tubing or clamp is checked.
• Incorrect needle placement or needle that won't advance through septum	• The device is reaccessed. • A home-care patient is taught to push down firmly on the noncoring needle device in the septum and to verify needle position by aspirating for blood return.
• Clot formation	• Patency is assessed by trying to flush the VAP while the patient changes position. • The physician is notified; an order is obtained for thrombolytic instillation. • The patient is taught to recognize clot formation, to notify the physician if it occurs, and to avoid forcibly flushing the VAP.
• Kinked catheter, catheter migration, or port rotation	• The physician is notified immediately. • The patient is told to notify the physician if he has difficulty using the VAP.
INABILITY TO PALPATE VAP	
• Deeply implanted port	• Portal chamber scar is noted. • Deep palpation technique is used. • Another nurse is asked to try locating the VAP. • A 1½" to 2" noncoring needle is used to gain access to the VAP.

- sterile 2" × 2" gauze pad and tape.

The syringes are labeled so the heparin and saline solution flushes aren't confused. Then these steps are followed:
- After shutting off the infusion, the extension set is clamped and the I.V. tubing removed.

Understanding complications of VAP therapy

This table lists common complications of vascular access port (VAP) therapy as well as their signs and symptoms, causes, nursing interventions, and preventive measures.

SIGNS AND SYMPTOMS	CAUSES
SITE INFECTION OR SKIN BREAKDOWN	
• Erythema, swelling, and warmth at the port site • Oozing or purulent drainage at the port site or VAP pocket • Fever	• Infected incision of VAP pocket • Poor postoperative healing
EXTRAVASATION	
• Burning sensation or swelling in subcutaneous tissue	• Needle dislodged into subcutaneous tissue • Needle incorrectly placed in VAP • Needle position not confirmed; needle pulled out of septum • Rupture of catheter along tunneled route
THROMBOSIS	
• Inability to flush port or administer infusion	• Frequent blood sampling • Infusion of packed red blood cells (RBCs)
FIBRIN SHEATH FORMATION	
• Blocked port and catheter lumen • Inability to flush port or administer infusion	• Adherence of platelets to catheter

- The syringe filled with saline solution is attached using sterile technique.
- The extension set is attached, the device flushed with the saline solution, and the saline solution syringe removed.

Nursing Interventions

- The site is assessed daily for redness; any drainage is noted.
- The physician is notified.
- Antibiotics, as prescribed, are administered.
- Warm soaks are applied for 20 minutes four times per day.

- The needle shouldn't be removed.
- The infusion is stopped.
- The physician is notified; the antidote is given.

- The physician is notified, and an order to give a thrombolytic according to facility policy is obtained. (If a radiologic device is used, radiology may be consulted).

- The physician is notified; the thrombolytic is prepared.

Prevention

- The patient should be taught to inspect for and report redness, swelling, drainage, or skin breakdown at the port site.

- The patient should be taught how to gain access to the device, verify placement of the device, and secure the needle before initiating the infusion.

- The VAP should be flushed thoroughly right after a blood sample is obtained.
- Packed RBCs should be given as a piggyback with saline solution; the system should be flushed with saline solution between units.

- The port should be used to infuse fluids and drugs, not to obtain blood samples.
- Only compatible substances should be given through the port.

■ The heparin syringe is attached, the VAP flushed with the heparin solution, and the extension set is clamped.

Removing the noncoring needle

After flushing the port with heparin solution, the noncoring needle is removed by following these steps:

- Gloves are put on.
- The gloved index and middle fingers from the nondominant hand are placed on either side of the port septum.
- The port is stabilized by pressing down with these two fingers, maintaining pressure until the needle is removed.
- With the gloved, dominant hand, the noncoring needle is grasped and pulled straight out of the port.
- A dressing is applied as indicated.
- If no more infusions are scheduled, the patient should be reminded that he'll need a heparin flush in 4 weeks.

Documenting

After removing the noncoring needle, the following is documented:

- removal of the infusion needle
- status of the site
- use of the heparin flush
- patient's tolerance of the procedure
- teaching efforts
- problems encountered and resolved.

4

ADMINISTERING I.V. DRUGS

Hospital patients receive about 40% of their drugs I.V. The drugs may be given by:
- direct injection
- intermittent infusion
- continuous infusion.

An I.V. drug may be ordered when:
- a patient needs a rapid therapeutic effect
- the drug can't be absorbed by the GI tract, either because it has a high molecular weight or is unstable in gastric juices
- the patient may receive nothing by mouth and an irritating drug would cause pain or tissue damage if given by I.M. or subcutaneous (subQ) injection
- a controlled administration rate is needed.

Benefits

Compared with the oral, subQ, and I.M. routes, the I.V. route has many advantages, including:
- rapid response
- effective absorption
- accurate titration
- less discomfort.

The I.V. route also provides an alternative to the oral route, such as when a patient is unconscious or uncooperative, or can take nothing by mouth.

In addition, if an adverse reaction occurs, I.V. drug delivery can be stopped immediately. With other routes, absorption would continue until the drug was physically removed by vomiting, gastric suctioning, or dialysis.

RAPID RESPONSE

I.V. drugs go directly into the patient's circulation, rapidly achieving therapeutic blood levels. This difference in absorption explains why, in drugs such as propranolol, I.V. doses are much smaller than oral doses.

EFFECTIVE ABSORPTION

Drug absorption covers the progress of a drug from the time it's given through the time it passes through the tissues, until it becomes available for use by the body. Absorption of subQ, I.M., and orally administered drugs may be problematic.

Absorption may be erratic with subQ and I.M. drug administration because the complex muscle and skin systems delay drug distribution. Giving drugs I.V. avoids this problem because the active drug reaches systemic circulation immediately, allowing the drug to achieve therapeutic levels quickly.

Some oral drugs are unstable in gastric juices and digestive enzymes, making absorption uncertain. Absorption problems also occur with oral drugs that are metabolized by the liver.

In the liver, significant amounts of the drug are processed and eliminated before they reach the bloodstream. This process — known as first-pass metabolism — may be so rapid and extensive (in the case of lidocaine, for example) that oral administration may not be practical.

ACCURATE TITRATION

Because gastric absorption isn't a factor with I.V. therapy, you can accurately titrate doses by adjusting the concentration of the infusing drug and the infusion rate.

LESSENED DISCOMFORT

I.V. administration prevents the pain and discomfort of I.M. or subQ injections. However, rapid delivery of some I.V. drugs can cause venous irritation. You may reduce venous irritation by further diluting an I.V. drug in a larger volume of diluent.

Risks

Like all administration routes, the I.V. route has certain risks. These include:
- solution and drug incompatibilities
- poor vascular access in some patients

- immediate adverse reactions.

INCOMPATIBILITY

To successfully mix a drug in a solution for infusion, two things need to be compatible: the drug and the diluent. If you aren't sure about the compatibility of a mixture, ask the pharmacist or check an I.V. compatibility chart. Most I.V. drugs are compatible with commonly used I.V. solutions. But when a solution is more complex, it will carry a greater risk of incompatibility.

Incompatibility problems are also common in mixtures containing:
- other electrolytes
- mannitol
- bicarbonate
- nutritional solutions.

Specific incompatibilities fall into three categories:
- physical
- chemical
- therapeutic. (See *Factors affecting drug compatibility,* page 152.)

A physical incompatibility (also called a pharmaceutical incompatibility) occurs more often with multiple additives.

Signs of physical incompatibility can be seen in the solution and include:
- precipitation
- haze
- gas bubbles
- cloudiness.

The presence of calcium in a solution (such as lactated Ringer's solution) usually increases the likelihood that a precipitate might form when the solution is mixed with another drug. Other physical incompatibilities occur as a result of drug degradation, such as the degradation of norepinephrine when added to sodium bicarbonate.

With chemical incompatibility, mixing two drugs alters the integrity and potency of active ingredients. When a drug loses more than 10% of its potency, it's considered incompatible with whatever caused the loss of potency. Decomposition of a drug indicates a chemical incompatibility. Factors commonly associated with chemical incompatibility include:
- drug concentration
- pH of the solution
- volume of solution used
- length of time the drugs are in contact with each other
- temperature
- light.

Factors affecting drug compatibility

Incompatibility is an undesirable chemical or physical reaction between a drug and a solution or between two or more drugs. The following factors can affect the compatibility of an I.V. drug or solution.

ORDER OF MIXING
Mixing order is a concern when you're adding more than one drug to an I.V. solution. Chemical changes occur after each drug is added. A drug that's compatible with the I.V. solution alone may be incompatible with the mixture of the I.V. solution and another drug. Changing the order in which the drugs are mixed may prevent incompatibility.

DRUG CONCENTRATION
The higher the drug concentration, the more likely an incompatibility will develop. Gently invert the container after adding each drug to evenly disperse it throughout the solution, preventing a high-concentration buildup. Do this before starting an infusion and before adding another drug to the container.

CONTACT TIME
The longer two or more drugs are together, the more likely an incompatibility will occur. For example, amikacin and acyclovir become incompatible when combined for 4 or more hours. You should know if two drugs are incompatible before deciding how to give them. Suppose, for example, the patient is receiving a continuous heparin infusion, and gentamicin sulfate is ordered. Because these two drugs have an immediate incompatibility, you shouldn't piggyback the gentamicin into the heparin solution. If you do, the patient won't receive a therapeutic dose of gentamicin.

TEMPERATURE
Higher temperatures promote chemical reactions. The higher the temperature of an admixture is, the greater the risk of incompatibility. For this reason, prepare the admixture immediately before administering it or refrigerate it until needed.

LIGHT
Prolonged exposure to light can affect the stability of certain drugs. Nitroprusside sodium and amphotericin B, for example, must be protected from light during administration to maintain their stability.

pH
Generally drugs and solutions that are to be mixed should have similar pH values to avoid incompatibility. The pH of each I.V. solution is listed on the manufacturer's label. You'll find the pH of each drug on the package insert.

The most common chemical incompatibility involves the reaction between acidic and alkaline drugs and solutions. For example, mixing a heparin solution with an intermittent aminoglycoside infusion commonly creates a chemical incompatibility, leading to such reactions as precipitate formation, color change, or gas bubbles.

Bright light, such as sunlight, may provide the energy needed for a chemical reaction. To avoid such a reaction, certain drugs must be protected from light. Examples of drugs that need protection from light when they're diluted are amphotericin B and sodium nitroprusside.

Therapeutic incompatibilities may occur when two or more drugs are given simultaneously. This may happen when a patient is prescribed two antibiotics — for example, chloramphenicol and penicillin. Chloramphenicol reportedly antagonizes penicillin's antibacterial action. Therefore, penicillin should be infused at least 1 hour before chloramphenicol.

POOR VASCULAR ACCESS

In an emergency, you may find that normally accessible veins have collapsed from vasoconstriction or hypovolemia. Venipuncture may also be difficult in patients who require frequent or prolonged I.V. therapy. You may find that they have developed small, scarred, inaccessible veins from repeated venipunctures or infusions of irritating drugs.

If peripheral venous access isn't possible, the prescriber may use a central vein, frequently the subclavian vein. If venipuncture isn't possible, drugs may be given I.M. or subQ. These routes can only be used if the volume to be infused is small and the drugs cause little or no tissue irritation.

ADVERSE REACTIONS

Because I.V. drugs quickly produce high blood levels, severe adverse reactions may occur immediately. The type of adverse reaction depends largely on the type of drug that's infused.

Hypersensitivity to I.V. drugs, although uncommon, can occur immediately or any time after administration. Keep cross-sensitivity in mind; if a patient is hypersensitive to a particular drug, he may be hypersensitive to chemically similar drugs. The most severe hypersensitivity reaction is anaphylaxis. Penicillin and its synthetic derivatives make up one of the drug families that are most likely to produce anaphylaxis. (See *Understanding anaphylaxis,* page 154.)

Your patient may suffer an adverse reaction to the preservative in a drug or I.V. solution. Sulfites, for example, can cause sensitivity reactions, particularly in patients with asthma. Large amounts of benzyl alcohol may cause seizures in neonates; all solutions given to neonates must be preservative-free.

Understanding anaphylaxis

Anaphylaxis is a dramatic, acute reaction marked by sudden onset of rapid, progressive urticaria and respiratory distress. A severe reaction may initiate vascular collapse, systemic shock, and even death.

Anaphylactic reactions result from systemic exposure to sensitizing drugs or other specific antigens. After exposure to an antigen, the immune system responds by producing specific immunoglobulin (Ig) antibodies in the lymph nodes. Helper T cells enhance the process. These antibodies, called IgE, then bind to membrane receptors located on mast cells (found throughout connective tissue, often near small blood vessels) and basophils.

When the body reencounters the antigen, the IgE antibodies or cross-linked IgE receptors recognize the antigen as foreign. This activates a series of cellular reactions that trigger *degranulation* – the release of chemical mediators (such as histamine, prostaglandins, and platelet-activating factor) from mast cell stores. IgG or IgM enters into the reaction and activates the release of complementary factors.

The most common anaphylaxis-causing antigen is penicillin. It causes a reaction in 1 to 4 out of every 10,000 patients. Penicillin is most likely to cause anaphylaxis after parenteral administration or prolonged therapy.

You may encounter patients who have an inherent inability to tolerate certain chemicals. They can experience another kind of adverse reaction, called an idiosyncratic reaction. For example, in a particular patient, a tranquilizer may cause excitation rather than sedation.

Calculating I.V. drug dosages

In many cases, you must calculate an ordered dosage and verify that the dosage is within the recommended range.

With some drugs (I.V. immune globulin, for instance), dosage is based on the patient's weight in kilograms. To convert a patient's weight from pounds to kilograms, simply divide the number of pounds by 2.2. (Remember, 2.2 lb = 1 kg.)

With other drugs (such as chemotherapeutic drugs), the dosage may be based on the patient's body surface area (BSA). One method for determining BSA is to use a nomogram. (See *Using a nomogram for children* and *Using a nomogram for adults,* page 156.)

Using a nomogram for children

To estimate a child's body surface area (BSA) with a nomogram, find the child's weight in the right column and his height in the left column. Mark these two points and draw a line between them. The point where the line intersects the surface area column in the middle gives you the BSA in square meters (m²).

On this nomogram, the child's height is 36″ (91.4 cm) and his weight is 55 lb (24.9 kg). A straight line drawn between the two columns intersects the center column at 0.8. That tells you that this patient's BSA is 0.8 m².

If the child is average size you can determine BSA from weight alone by using the boxed area.

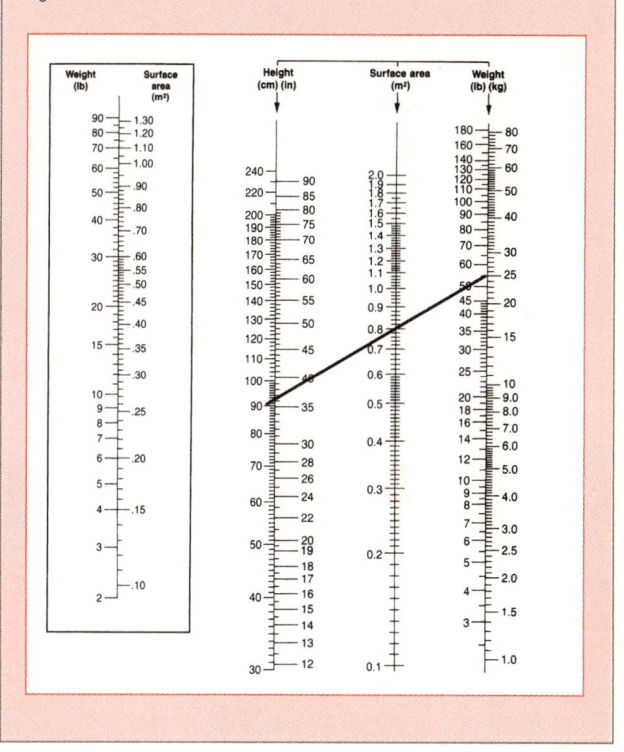

Using a nomogram for adults

To estimate an adult's body surface area (BSA) with a nomogram, find the patient's weight in the right column and his height in the left column. Mark these two points and draw a line between them. The point where the line intersects the middle column gives you the BSA in square meters (m²).

On this nomogram, the patient's height is 5'3" (160 cm) and her weight is 110 lb (49.9 kg). A straight line drawn between the two columns intersects the center column at 1.50. That tells you this patient's BSA is 1.5 m².

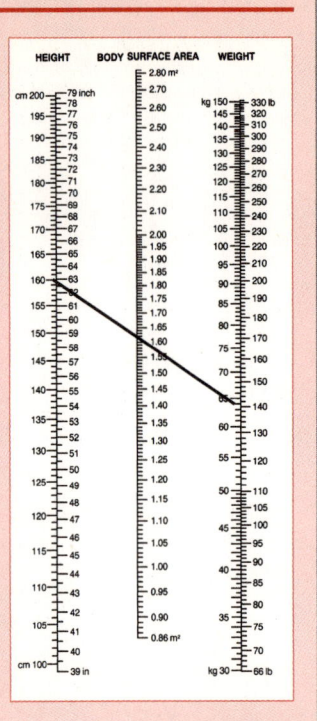

Calculating infusion rates

Typically, an order for an I.V. drug gives the number of milliliters to infuse over a specified period. For instance, an order may call for 1,000 ml of dextrose 5% in half-normal saline solution every 8 hours.

To make sure you deliver the drug solution correctly, you need to determine how many milliliters to give in 1 hour. To do this divide the total volume of the infusion by the number of hours the infusion will take. In this case, divide 1,000 ml by 8 hours to determine that you must give 125 ml/hour.

ADDITIONAL ORDERS

Additional I.V. orders affect your calculations. Suppose the patient who's receiving 1,000 ml of dextrose 5% in half-normal saline solution every 8 hours also needs to receive 80 mg gentamicin once every 8 hours by intermittent infusion. There are two possible ways to handle this:

- After determining that the patient can tolerate the extra volume, you may simply incorporate the antibiotic fluid into the total daily intake.
- After determining that gentamicin and the primary infusate (dextrose 5% in half-normal saline solution) are compatible, you may recalculate the infusion rate for the primary infusion after the antibiotic has been given.

To recalculate the infusion rate for the previous example, use these two steps:

- Subtract the time needed to give the gentamicin from the total time period. For example, if you administer the gentamicin over 1 hour, there are 7 hours left to give the primary solution.
- Divide 1,000 by 7 to find that you must deliver the primary solution at a rate of 143 ml/hour.

EQUIPMENT CONSIDERATIONS

Your calculations may also depend on the delivery equipment. If you're using an infusion pump, simply set the dial for the desired milliliters per hour rate. However, if you're using an administration set, you have to convert milliliters per hour to drops per minute (gtt/minute).

To convert milliliters per hour to drops per minute, you must know the number of drops per milliliter that the particular I.V. tubing delivers. Microdrip tubing delivers 60 gtt/ml, but macrodrip tubing varies. To find drops per milliliter information, check the product wrapper or box; then use this formula:

$$\text{drip rate in drops/ml} = \frac{\text{total milliliters}}{\text{total minutes}} \times \text{drop factor in drops/minute}$$

Nurse practice act restrictions

The scope of practice about the administration of I.V. drugs for LPNs varies widely from state to state. In many states it isn't allowed; in others, LPNs may not give titrated drugs and I.V push but can give continuous infusions. You'll need to check your state's nurse practice act as well as your facility policy to determine if giving I.V. drugs is in your scope of practice. If it is in your scope, check for restrictions on the types of drugs you can give and the ways that you can give them.

Preparing drugs

Most I.V. drug solutions are prepared in the pharmacy by pharmacists or pharmacy technicians. However, you may have to prepare I.V. drug solutions yourself. When preparing a drug for I.V. administration, be sure to take some basic safety measures.

- Maintain sterile technique. Always wash your hands before mixing, and avoid contaminating any part of the vial, ampule, syringe, needle, or container that must remain sterile. When you're inserting the needle into the vial and withdrawing it, make sure the needle tip doesn't touch any part of the vial that isn't sterile. Make sure you don't inadvertently puncture your finger; to keep your hands steady, brace one against the other while you're inserting and withdrawing the needle.
- When drawing up the drug before adding it to the primary solution, make sure you use a syringe that's large enough to hold the entire dose. The needle should be at least 1″ long to penetrate the inner seal of the port on an I.V. bag. In many facilities, practitioners use a 5-micron filter needle for mixing drug powder or withdrawing drugs from glass ampules. This needle is then removed, a sterile 1″ needle is attached to the syringe, and the drug is then admixed. (See *Keep it safe*.)
- In many facilities, premixed doses are drawn up into a syringe in the pharmacy. A 24-hour supply is delivered to the nursing unit, where the drug is stored in a refrigerator. The nurse then gives the dose using a syringe pump that delivers the drug over time.

RECONSTITUTING POWDERED DRUGS

Many I.V. drugs are supplied in powder form and have to be reconstituted with liquid diluents.

Common diluents include:
- normal saline solution
- sterile water for injection
- dextrose 5% in water.

Keep it safe

Make sure you follow a few basic tips to ensure safety when you administer I.V. drugs.

CHECK IT OUT
Check the expiration date on the drug and the diluent, and look for any special diluent requirements. Note whether the drug requires filtration. Inspect the drug, diluent, and solution for particles and cloudiness. After reconstitution, again check for visible signs of incompatibility in the admixture. Remember, incompatibility is more likely with drugs or I.V. solutions that have a high or low pH. Most drugs are moderately acidic, but some are alkaline, including heparin, aminophylline, ampicillin sodium, and sodium bicarbonate.

MIXING IN A MINIBAG
If you're mixing a drug in a minibag or minibottle of normal saline solution or dextrose 5% in water, you may be able to use the solution in the minicontainer as the diluent. However, be sure to inspect it and discard any solution that appears cloudy or contains particles. Some solutions change color after several hours. If you aren't sure whether to use a discolored solution, ask the pharmacist.

Note the manufacturer's instructions about the right type or amount of diluent. Some drugs should be reconstituted with diluents that contain preservatives. (See *Reconstituting powdered drugs*, page 160.)

Some drugs come in double-chambered vials that contain powder in the lower chamber and a diluent in the upper one. To combine the contents, press the rubber stopper on top of the vial to dislodge the rubber plug separating the compartments. The diluent then mixes with the drug in the bottom chamber.

DILUTING LIQUID DRUGS

A liquid drug may be packed in:
- single-dose ampules or vials
- multidose vials
- prefilled syringes
- disposable cartridges.

Liquid drugs don't need reconstitution, but they usually require further dilution.

There are several methods you can use to add a drug to an I.V. container. Additive vials of a drug can be attached directly to ad-

Reconstituting powdered drugs

To safely reconstitute powdered drugs, gather the needed equipment and then follow these step-by-step guidelines.

DRAW UP AND CLEAN
First you need to:
- draw up the amount and type of diluent specified by the manufacturer
- clean the rubber stopper of the drug vial with an alcohol swab using sterile technique.

INSERT, INJECT, AND MIX
When the diluent is drawn up and the stopper is clean, you can insert, inject, and mix:
- Insert the needle connected to the syringe of diluent into the stopper at a 45- to 60-degree angle. Angling the needle minimizes coring or breaking off rubber pieces, which would then float inside the vial.
- Inject the diluent.
- Mix thoroughly by gently inverting the vial. If the drug doesn't dissolve within a few seconds, let it stand for 10 to 30 minutes. If necessary, invert the vial several times to dissolve the drug. Don't shake vigorously (unless directed) because some drugs may froth.

---

ministration tubing. If the vial contains a drug powder, first reconstitute it. Then you can infuse the drug solution directly from the vial, using dedicated vented tubing. (See *Adding a drug to an I.V. container.*)

LABELING SOLUTION CONTAINERS
A container prepared in the pharmacy has a label showing:
- patient's full name
- patient's room number
- date
- name and amount of the I.V. solution and drugs
- vital information such as the infusion rate.

If you prepare the drug solution, be sure to label the container with the same information provided by the pharmacy. Also note the date and time you mixed the drug solution and sign or initial the label. Make sure your label doesn't cover the manufacturer's label. If you use a time strip, label it with the patient's name and room number and the infusion rate (in milliliters per hour, drops per minute, or both).

> **BEST PRACTICE**
>
> ## Adding a drug to an I.V. container
>
> To add a drug to an I.V. container, use the following step-by-step techniques for safe mixing.
>
> ### ADDING TO AN I.V. BOTTLE
> To add a drug to an I.V. bottle, first clean the rubber stopper or latex diaphragm with alcohol. Then insert the 19G or 20G needle of the drug-filled syringe into the center of the stopper or diaphragm and inject the drug. Next, invert the bottle at least twice to ensure thorough mixing. Finally, remove the latex diaphragm and insert the administration spike.
>
> ### ADDING TO AN I.V. BAG
> To add a drug to a plastic I.V. bag, insert the needle of the medication-filled syringe into the clean latex medication port and inject the drug. (The needle should be 19G or 20G and 1" long; a short needle won't pierce the inner port seal, and a small-volume additive, such as insulin, will remain in the port.) After injecting the drug, grasp the top and bottom of the bag and quickly invert it twice. Don't squeeze or shake the bag.
>
> ### ADDING TO AN INFUSING SOLUTION
> If you have a choice, don't add a drug to an I.V. solution that's already infusing because of the risk of altering the drug concentration. However, if you must add a drug, make sure the primary solution container has enough solution to provide adequate dilution. To add the drug, clamp the I.V. tubing and take down the container. Then with the container upright, add the drug.
>
> If you're adding the drug to a bottle, clean the rubber stopper with an alcohol swab, insert the needle through the stopper, and inject the drug. If you're adding the drug to an I.V. bag, clean the rubber injection port with an alcohol swab before you inject the drug.
>
> ### *MIX WELL*
> After injecting the drug into the container, invert it several times to ensure thorough mixing and prevent a bolus effect.

Selecting the equipment

When choosing the equipment you'll use to administer I.V. drugs, you need to consider several factors. For example, which drug has been prescribed? What's the ordered infusion rate? Is your patient an adult or a child? Which equipment options are available? Your selection will depend on the answers to these and many other questions. (See *Choosing the right equipment*, pages 162 and 163.)

Choosing the right equipment

Consider the following questions to help you choose equipment that's appropriate for administering any drug.

PUMP
Do you need a pump to deliver a particular drug? Health care facilities usually have policies regarding the use of these devices. Pumps, most of which still require specific administration sets, are commonly used when you need a precise or very low infusion rate. They're also used when you're administering fluids or admixtures through a central venous catheter.

INFUSION RATE
What's the ordered infusion rate and what's your facility's policy on using macrodrip and microdrip tubing? Many policies require microdrip tubing when the infusion rate is less than 63 ml/hour.

INTERMITTENT INFUSIONS
Is the patient going to receive intermittent drug infusions as well as the primary drug solution? If so, you may need a primary tubing that has an injection port close to the drip chamber and a backcheck valve that will automatically shut off the primary solution when the secondary solution is infusing.

SIMULTANEOUS INFUSIONS
Is the patient going to receive a simultaneous infusion of a secondary drug solution? If so, first make sure the drugs are compatible, then choose tubing that has an injection port close to the venipuncture device so you don't have to stop the primary infusion.

SPECIAL TUBING
Does the drug solution require special tubing? Tubing without polyvinyl chloride is recommended for certain drugs, such as nitroglycerin or paclitaxel (Taxol).

GLASS OR PLASTIC
Is the solution container made of glass or plastic? If you're using a glass container, you need vented I.V. tubing. Use nonvented tubing for a collapsible plastic bag.

INFANT OR SMALL CHILD
Is the patient an infant or a small child? Many facilities have policies that permit only volume-control sets for such patients. These devices limit the volume available to the patient and decrease the risk of inadvertent fluid overload.

(continued)

Choosing the right equipment (continued)

NEEDLE-FREE

Most facilities use needleless systems. You can piggyback drugs or additional I.V. solutions into a primary line without using a needle. Instead, a system is used that consists of a blunt-tipped device and a rubber injection port, as shown at right. These items are called *access devices* or *adaptation devices*. The port may be part of a special administration set or an adapter for existing administration sets. This rubber injection port has a preestablished slit that can open and reseal immediately.

A needleless system greatly reduces the risk of accidental needle-stick injuries, but it can't eliminate all such injuries because this system can't be used to perform venipunctures.

Needleless systems can be used to obtain blood for blood gas analysis and other laboratory tests.

Indwelling lines, such as A-lines or central lines, can be adapted for use with the needleless system. It's possible to adapt a line for use with needleless systems with replaceable injection ports.

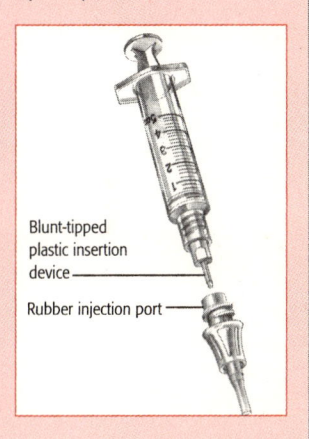

Blunt-tipped plastic insertion device

Rubber injection port

Preparing the patient

Before you give an I.V. drug by any method, take time to properly prepare the patient and the drug. Follow these steps:

- Confirm the patient's identity using two patient identifiers (not the patient's room number). (See *Remember the five rights,* page 164.)
- Make sure you know some key information about the drug you're giving. For instance, you should know the normal dosage, expected effects, adverse reactions, contraindications, and drug interactions. If you're unfamiliar with the drug and don't have access to the drug package insert or a drug reference book, ask your pharmacist any drug-related questions.
- Follow the Centers for Disease Control and Prevention guidelines to protect yourself and the patient from blood-borne pathogens

> **BEST PRACTICE**
>
> ## Remember the five rights
>
> Before you administer an I.V. drug to a patient, make sure that you check the five rights:
> - right drug
> - right patient
> - right time
> - right dosage
> - right route.
>
> **THERE'S ACTUALLY A SIXTH RIGHT**
> At the same time, make sure that the patient understands the drug he will receive and knows he has the right to refuse it.

and infection. These guidelines require you to wear gloves (and possibly a gown and mask) when exposed to body fluids.

Infusion methods

I.V. drugs can be given by three methods:
- direct injection
- intermittent infusion
- continuous infusion.

You may also give an I.V. drug using a specialized device such as a patient-controlled analgesia (PCA) electronic infusion device. (See *Comparing administration methods,* pages 165 to 167.)

DIRECT INJECTION

Check your state's nurse practice act and facility policy to determine if giving I.V. drugs through direct injection is in your scope of practice. In many states it isn't allowed. In others, it's allowed after the LPN has had some experience and special training.

Direct injection can be used to deliver a single dose (bolus) or intermittent multiple doses. Commonly called an I.V. push, a direct injection can be given two ways: directly into a vein or through an existing infusion line. Direct injection may cause localized site complications. This method exerts more pressure on the vein than other methods, posing a greater risk of infiltration in patients with fragile veins.

Most drugs must be given over a specific period of time when using direct injection. To avoid speed shock, don't give any drug in

Comparing administration methods

This table gives you the indications, advantages, and disadvantages of common I.V. administration methods.

METHODS AND INDICATIONS	ADVANTAGES	DISADVANTAGES
DIRECT INJECTION		
INTO A VEIN (NO INFUSION LINE) • When a nonvesicant drug with low risk of immediate adverse reaction is required for a patient with no other I.V. needs (for example, an outpatient requiring I.V. contrast injections for radiologic examinations or a cancer patient receiving chemotherapeutic agents)	• Eliminates the risk of complications from an indwelling venipuncture device • Eliminates the inconvenience of an indwelling venipuncture device	• Can only be given by a physician or certified nurse • Requires venipuncture, which can cause patient anxiety • Requires two syringes—one to administer the medication and one to flush the vein after administration • Risk of infiltration from steel needle • Drug can't be diluted and delivery can't be interrupted if irritation occurs • Carries risk of clotting with administration of a drug over a long period and with a small volume
THROUGH EXISTING INFUSION LINE • When a drug is incompatible with the I.V. solution and must be given as bolus injection • When a patient requires immediate high blood levels (for example, regular insulin, dextrose 50%, atropine, and antihistamines) • In emergencies, for immediate drug effect	• Doesn't require time or authorization to perform venipuncture because the vein is already accessed • Doesn't require a needle puncture, which can cause patient anxiety • Allows the use of I.V. solution to test the patency of the venipuncture device before drug administration • Allows continued venous access in case of adverse reactions	• Carries the same inconveniences and risk of complications associated with indwelling venipuncture device (such as infection, infiltration, and pain)

(continued)

Comparing administration methods (*continued*)

METHODS AND INDICATIONS	ADVANTAGES	DISADVANTAGES
INTERMITTENT INFUSION		
PIGGYBACK METHOD • Commonly used with drugs given over short periods at varying intervals (for example, antibiotics and gastric-secretion inhibitors)	• Avoids multiple needle injections required by I.M. route • Permits repeated administration of drugs through a single I.V. site • Provides high drug blood levels for short periods without causing drug toxicity	• May cause periods when the drug blood level becomes too low to be clinically effective (for example, when peak and trough times aren't considered in the medication order)
SALINE LOCK • When a patient requires constant venous access but not a continuous infusion	• Provides venous access for patients with fluid restrictions • Provides better patient mobility between doses • Preserves veins by reducing venipunctures • Lowers cost if used with a limited number of drugs	• Requires close monitoring during administration so the device can be flushed on completion
VOLUME-CONTROL SET • When a patient requires a low volume of fluid	• Requires only one large-volume container • Prevents fluid overload from a runaway infusion • Allows the chamber to be reused	• High cost • Carries a high risk of contamination • If there is no membrane to block air passage when empty, flow clamp must be closed when the set empties
CONTINUOUS INFUSION		
THROUGH PRIMARY LINE • To maintain continuous serum levels, if the infusion isn't likely to be stopped abruptly	• Maintains steady serum levels • Presents less risk of rapid shock and vein irritation because of a large volume of fluid diluting the drug	• Risk of incompatibility increases with drug contact time • Restricts patient mobility • Carries an increased risk of infiltration

Comparing administration methods *(continued)*

METHODS AND INDICATIONS	ADVANTAGES	DISADVANTAGES

CONTINUOUS INFUSION *(continued)*

THROUGH SECONDARY LINE
- When a patient requires continuous infusion of two or more compatible admixtures administered at different rates
- When there's a significant chance of abruptly stopping one admixture without infusing the remaining drug in I.V. tubing

- Allows primary infusion and each secondary infusion to be given at different rates
- Allows primary line to be totally shut off and kept on stand-by to maintain venous access in case secondary line must be abruptly stopped
- Short contact time before infusion may allow the administration of incompatible admixtures — something not possible with long contact time

- Can't be used for drugs with immediate incompatibility
- Carries an increased risk of vein irritation or phlebitis from an increased number of drugs
- Use of multiple I.V. systems (for example, primary lines with secondary lines attached), especially with electronic pumps, can create physical barriers to patient care and limit patient mobility

---

less than 1 minute unless the order directs you to do so or the patient is in cardiac or respiratory arrest.

To avoid decreased drug tolerance, slower injection times or greater drug dilution may be required if your patient has:
- systemic edema
- pulmonary congestion
- decreased cardiac output
- reduced urine output, renal flow, or glomerular filtration rate.

Certain drugs metabolize quickly and must be given quickly to achieve the desired effect. One such drug is adenosine, used to treat supraventricular tachycardia.

Injection into a vein

If your state nurse practice act and facility policy allow you to inject a drug directly into a vein, you need these supplies:
- winged small-vein needle
- syringe with drug
- 3-ml syringe filled with saline solution
- povidone-iodine or alcohol swab

Injecting a drug directly into a vein

Not all states allow LPNs to perform this procedure. Therefore, first check with your state nurse practice act. Then after assembling your equipment, follow the steps outlined here to safely and accurately inject a drug directly into a vein.

APPLY, CONNECT, SELECT, WITHDRAW
Begin with these steps:
- Apply the tourniquet and clean the I.V. site with a povidone-iodine or alcohol swab.
- Connect the syringe with medication to the small-vein needle and push the plunger to expel the air.
- Select the largest suitable vein to allow for rapid dilution. Put on gloves and insert the needle in the vein with the bevel up.
- Withdraw a small amount of blood to confirm needle placement.

RELEASE, SECURE, INJECT, ASPIRATE
When you're certain the needle is properly placed, proceed with these steps:
- Release the tourniquet.
- Place a short narrow strip of tape or a transparent dressing over each needle wing to secure the device during administration.
- Inject the drug at an even rate, as ordered.
- Gently aspirate the plunger at frequent intervals to reconfirm needle placement and ensure the delivery of all drug.

OBSERVE, DISCONNECT, REMOVE, DISPOSE
After the drug is injected:
- Observe the patient for signs of adverse reactions (during and after the injection).
- Disconnect the drug syringe from the small-vein needle. Attach the syringe filled with saline to the needle and flush the device to ensure the complete delivery of all drug.
- Remove the venipuncture device and immediately place a sterile pressure dressing over the I.V. site.
- Dispose of contaminated hazardous equipment.

SOMETHING TO CONSIDER
If the patient needs further I.V. therapy – or if the drug can cause an immediate adverse reaction – consider getting an order for an indwelling access device.

- tourniquet
- gloves
- tape
- sterile pressure dressing.

Use the winged needle for I.V. push because it can be inserted quickly and easily. You also need dressing materials to apply to the venipuncture site after administration and a nonpermeable container in which to discard contaminated equipment. (See *Injecting a drug directly into a vein.*)

> ### Injecting a drug into an existing line
>
> If your state nurse practice act or facility policy allows you to perform this procedure, assemble the equipment and then follow the step-by-step technique described here to inject a drug safely into an existing line.
>
> **CHECK, FLUSH, INVERT, CLEAN**
> Begin with these steps:
> - Check the I.V. site for redness, tenderness, edema, or leakage. If you detect any of these signs of complications, change the site before you administer the drug.
> - If the new drug and the existing infusate are compatible, keep the infusion running. If the drug isn't compatible with the infusate but is compatible with saline solution, use a saline-filled syringe to flush the line before injecting the drug.
> - Invert the syringe and gently push the plunger to remove all air.
> - Using an alcohol swab, clean the rubber cap of the injection port closest to the venous access device.
>
> **STABILIZE, INJECT, OBSERVE, WITHDRAW**
> After completing initial preparations, continue with these steps:
> - Stabilize the injection port with one hand and insert the needleless device (or needle) through the center of the rubber cap. Don't force the insertion. If you meet resistance, position the needle or needleless device at a different angle.
> - Inject the drug at an even rate. Never inject so fast that you stop the primary infusion or allow the drug to flow back into the tubing.
> - Observe the patient for signs of a reaction during and after the injection.
> - Withdraw the needleless device (or needle) and reestablish the desired flow rate.

Injection into an existing line

To give an injection directly into the injection port of an existing line, you need these supplies:
- drug
- syringe with a needleless system (or a 22G 1″ needle if a needleless system isn't available)
- alcohol swab
- saline-filled syringe for flushing. (See *Injecting a drug into an existing line.*)

INTERMITTENT INFUSION

The most common and flexible method of giving an I.V. drug is intermittent infusion. In this method, a drug is given over a specified period at varying intervals. This helps to maintain and monitor a therapeutic level. A small volume (1 to 250 ml) may be delivered over several minutes or a few hours.

Secondary line

If your state nurse practice act or facility policy allow you to infuse a drug through a secondary line, you need these supplies:
- drug in the unit-dose container
- secondary infusion tubing
- needleless device (or a 22G 1″ needle if a needleless device isn't available)
- alcohol swab
- 1″ adhesive tape
- extension hook for the primary container.

You can deliver an intermittent infusion through a piggyback line that's connected to the primary line through a port, a saline lock, or a volume-control set.

The primary line should have a side Y-port with a backcheck valve that stops the flow from the primary line during drug infusion and resumes the primary flow after infusion. (See *Setting up a piggyback set*.)

To perform the procedure, follow these steps:
- Check the I.V. site for infiltration, phlebitis, or infection.
- Check the primary infusion line for patency.
- Make sure that the drug to be piggybacked is compatible with the primary infusion.
- Hang the bag on the I.V. pole.
- Close the flow clamp on the secondary tubing, remove the covers to the container and tubing spike, and insert the spike firmly into the container port.
- Secure the needle or needleless device to the secondary tubing. Then using an alcohol swab, clean the injection port on the primary tubing.
- Remove the cover from the secondary tubing and make sure the needle or needleless device is secure. When using a needle, secure it with tape to prevent dislodgment. Insert the full length of the device into the center of the injection port.
- Lower the primary infusion with the supplied extension hook below the level of the secondary container, open the flow clamp of the secondary set, and allow the drug to infuse as prescribed.

Because the secondary container hangs higher than the primary container, fluid flowing from the secondary creates pressure on the backcheck valve and completely shuts off fluid flow from the primary. After the secondary infusion is completed, the primary fluid automatically flows again. When this happens, close the clamp on the secondary tubing and readjust the infusion rate of the primary infusion.

Setting up a piggyback set

Used only for intermittent drug infusions, a piggyback set includes a secondary container (a small I.V. bag or bottle) and short tubing with a drip chamber. To use it, connect the piggyback set to a primary line with a Y-port (or piggyback port), as shown. You must use an extension hook to position the primary I.V. container below the secondary container.

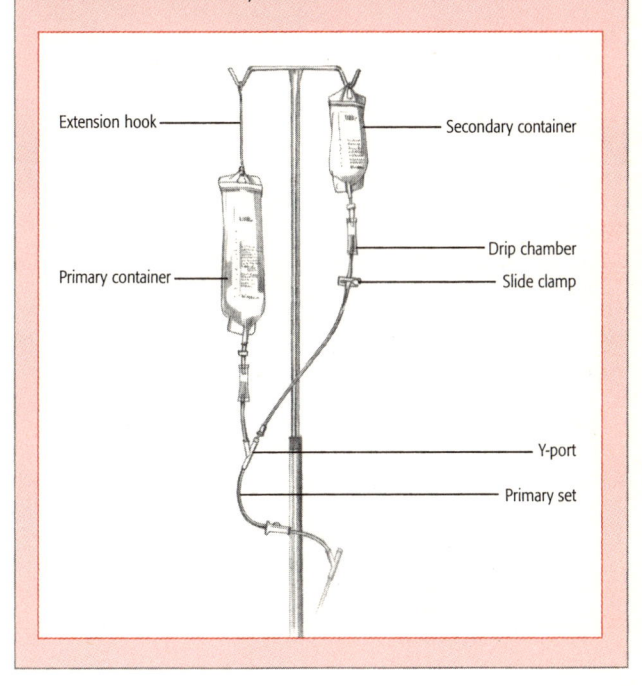

Labels: Extension hook, Primary container, Secondary container, Drip chamber, Slide clamp, Y-port, Primary set

If the primary tubing doesn't have a backcheck valve, you must clamp the primary line; you don't need to lower the primary container. Remember to open the primary clamp when the piggyback infusion is completed. Otherwise the infusion device may clog and the patient may not receive the volume of I.V. fluid prescribed.

Many drugs pose a high risk of phlebitis. Be sure to check the I.V. site carefully before giving each dose. If necessary, change the site before you give the drug.

Using a saline lock

Use the following step-by-step guidelines to safely administer a drug using a saline lock.

ATTACH, SECURE, CLEAN, STABILIZE
After assembling the equipment, begin with these steps:
- Attach the minibag to the administration set and prime the tubing with the drug solution.
- Secure the needleless device to the I.V. tubing device and prime the needleless device with the drug solution.
- Using an alcohol swab, clean the cap on the saline lock.
- Stabilize the saline lock with the thumb and index finger of your nondominant hand, as shown below right.

INSERT, FLUSH, SECURE, INFUSE
When the saline lock is stabilized continue with these steps:
- Insert the needleless device of one of the syringes containing flush solution into the center of the injection cap. Don't force it; if you feel resistance, insert the device at a different angle. Pull back on the plunger slightly and watch for blood return. If blood appears begin to slowly inject the flush solution. If you feel resistance or if the patient complains of pain or discomfort stop immediately because the venous access device should be replaced.
- If you don't feel resistance watch for signs of infiltration as you slowly inject the flush solution. If you note signs of infiltration remove the infusion device and insert a new device in a new location; if you don't note any signs you're ready to give the medication.
- Insert the needleless device attached to the administration set into the saline lock.
- Regulate the drip rate and infuse the drug.

CLOSE AND CLEAN
To stop the infusion:
- Close the I.V. flow clamp and withdraw the needleless device.
- Clean the injection cap and flush the saline lock again.

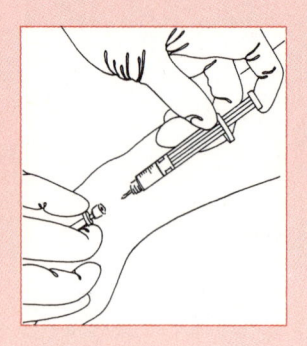

Saline lock

For intermittent I.V. drug infusion with a saline lock or intermittent device, you need these supplies:
- drug solution in its container
- administration set

Hints for handling a saline lock

Here are helpful hints for using a saline lock.

CHECK CAREFULLY
Before accessing the lock, check the I.V. site carefully and change it if necessary.

LARGE ENOUGH AND SMALL ENOUGH
Access the intermittent cap with a needleless device (or a needle if a needleless device isn't available) of the appropriate gauge and length.

AVOIDING MOVEMENT
When the injection cap serves as a saline lock, stabilize the cap while accessing and removing the I.V. tubing and needle or needleless device to prevent movement at the insertion site. Movement increases the risks of phlebitis and catheter dislodgment.

BE PRESENT
You must be present when the infusion runs out so you can disconnect the tubing and flush the device. Otherwise, clots will form in the saline lock.

EVERY 6 TO 24 HOURS
Flush the device after each use and as needed with the volume of solution recommended by facility policy. The flush solution is typically saline. Flushing may be required every 6 to 24 hours depending on facility policy.

TIME FOR NEW TUBING
Follow your facility's policy for tubing changes. If you have to reconnect used tubing, make sure the tubing needle adapter hasn't been contaminated. Always use a sterile needleless device.

GIVING DRUGS
You can also give a drug by direct injection through a saline lock. In this case, flush the saline lock, inject the drug, and flush the saline lock again.

- needleless device (or a 20G 1″ needle if a needleless device isn't available)
- alcohol swab.

You also need two 3-ml syringes filled with saline flush solution each connected to a needleless device. (See *Using a saline lock*, and *Hints for handling a saline lock*.)

Volume-control set

You can use a volume-control set as either a primary or secondary line. When using a volume-control set as a primary line gather these supplies:

- I.V. solution

Adding to a volume-control set

After wiping the injection port with an alcohol swab, inject the drug with a syringe, as shown below.

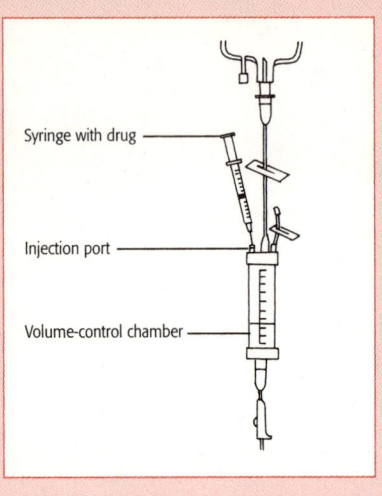

- Syringe with drug
- Injection port
- Volume-control chamber

- drug in a syringe with a needleless device (or a 20G 1" needle if a needleless device isn't available)
- alcohol swabs
- a label.

When using a volume-control set as a secondary line gather these supplies:
- I.V. solution
- adhesive tape (for piggybacking)
- drug in a syringe with a needleless device
- alcohol swabs
- a label.

To perform the procedure, follow these steps:
- Check the I.V. line for patency and the I.V. site for signs of infiltration or phlebitis.
- If you're using the volume-control set as a primary line, prime the tubing with the I.V. solution. Insert the adapter of the set into the venipuncture device or saline lock.

Tips for adding drugs

When adding medications to a volume-control set, check for an immediately visible incompatibility – especially if you're using multiple lines. Also follow these tips.

TANGLES
To prevent confusion when using multiple secondary lines, don't let them become tangled. Tag the lines below the drip chamber and at the connection site to the primary line. This clearly identifies the source and tubing connection for each drug.

PUMPS
When possible, use a pump to achieve more accurate dosage control. Put a time strip on the secondary container to help monitor the administration rate.

SECURE, PATENT, AND FIRMLY STABLE
Maintain a secure, patent infusion device. To avoid interrupting drug therapy when you change the I.V. site, establish the new site before disconnecting the old one. Firmly stabilize the connection to the primary tubing with tape or a locking device to prevent dislodgment.

- If you're using the volume-control set as a secondary line, attach the needleless device to the adapter on the set and prime the tubing and needle with the I.V. solution. Wipe the injection site on the primary tubing with an alcohol swab, and insert the needleless device into the injection port. Needleless devices have a locking mechanism.
- To add drug to the chamber, wipe the injection port on the volume-control set with an alcohol swab and inject the drug. (See *Adding to a volume-control set*, and *Tips for adding drugs*.)
- Place a label on the chamber indicating the drug, dose, time, and date. Don't write directly on the chamber with ink (the plastic can absorb the ink). Don't place the label over the numbers of the chamber. Open the upper clamp; fill the fluid chamber with the prescribed amount of solution to dilute the drug. Close the clamp. Gently rotate the chamber to mix the drug and the solution.
- If you're using the volume-control set as a secondary line, either stop the primary infusion or set a low infusion rate so the line will be open when the secondary infusion is completed. Open the lower clamp of the volume-control set and adjust the infusion rate.

- After the infusion is completed and if the patient can tolerate the extra fluid, open the upper clamp and let 10 ml of I.V. solution flow into the chamber and through the tubing to flush it and complete delivery of the drug to the patient.
- If you're using the volume-control set as a secondary line, close the lower clamp and reset the infusion rate on the primary line. If you're using the set as a primary line, close the lower clamp, refill the chamber to the prescribed amount of primary solution, and restart the infusion.
- Instead of using the volume-control set as a primary line, you can mix the drug in the primary solution, then use the volume-control chamber to closely regulate the amount of fluid and the drug dosage the patient receives.

If you're using a volume-control set with a membrane for intermittent drug administration, fill the chamber with fluid before adding the drug. This prevents the membrane from becoming sticky and difficult to operate. Be sure to read the manufacturer's instructions for priming a volume-control set.

The infusion stops when the fluid chamber is empty. If the set doesn't have a membrane or shut-off valve, refill the fluid chamber quickly to prevent air from filling the set.

CONTINUOUS INFUSION

A continuous infusion allows you to carefully regulate drug delivery over a prolonged period. A continuous infusion may be given through a peripheral or central venous line. Sometimes, before you start a continuous infusion, a loading dose is given to achieve a peak level quickly.

A continuous infusion enhances the effectiveness of some drugs, such as insulin and heparin. Delivery of these drugs is commonly regulated with an I.V. pump.

Primary line

To give a continuous infusion through a primary line, you need these supplies:
- prescribed drug in I.V. solution
- administration set
- gloves.

To ensure proper infusion use an infusion pump and make sure you have the correct administration set for the pump. Prepare to give a continuous infusion with these steps:
- Make sure the I.V. solution container is labeled with the name and dosage of the drug.

Infusion methods

- Attach the administration set to the solution container and prime the tubing with the I.V. solution.
- Attach the administration set to the pump, if needed.
- Perform or assist with the venipuncture, if needed.

To begin the infusion, follow these steps:
- Put on gloves.
- Remove the protective cap at the end of the administration set.
- Attach the set to the catheter.
- Begin the infusion and regulate the flow to the ordered rate. Remember to frequently monitor the patient and the infusion rate.
- When the infusion is completed, hang another solution container or change solutions, if needed.

Maintain accurate intake and output records and be alert for excessive fluid retention and fluid overload. Weigh the patient daily, wearing the same clothes and at the same time of day. When a patient receives small amounts hourly, his total daily volume can be excessive without any obvious signs.

Remember, too, that giving a large volume of fluid can seriously change a patient's electrolyte levels. Make sure you check the patient's laboratory results to make sure his electrolyte levels stay within normal limits.

Check the infusion rate at regular intervals to ensure that the drug is delivered correctly. Check I.V. sites frequently for signs of complications. If you note tenderness, redness, swelling, or leakage, stop the infusion and treat the site according to facility policy. Restart the infusion in another vein.

Secondary line

To give a continuous infusion through a secondary line, make sure you have these supplies:
- prescribed drug in I.V. solution
- administration set
- needleless device (or a 20G 1″ needle if a needleless device isn't available)
- alcohol swabs
- 1″ adhesive tape.

You may also need an infusion pump. If so, make sure you have the correct administration set for the pump. (See *Infusing medication through a secondary line,* page 178.)

After you give a drug I.V., always document the procedure. (See *Documenting I.V. drug administration,* page 179.)

> ### Infusing medication through a secondary line
>
> If your state nurse practice act or facility policy allows, follow the step-by-step technique here to safely administer medication through a secondary line.
>
> **ATTACH, PRIME, LABEL, CLEAN**
> After assembling the necessary equipment, begin with these steps:
> - Attach the administration set to the solution container and prime the tubing with the I.V. solution. If appropriate, attach the administration set to the pump.
> - Secure the needleless device – or, if one isn't available, a 22G 1" needle – to the administration set and prime the device with the I.V. solution.
> - Place labels with the name of the drug under the drip chamber and at the end of the tubing.
> - Clean the injection port on the primary tubing with an alcohol swab.
>
> **INSERT, ADJUST, MONITOR, REMOVE**
> When you have ensured that the injection port is clean, continue with these steps:
> - Insert the full length of the needleless adapter into the center of the injection port. If a needleless device isn't available and you must use a needle, secure the needle with tape to prevent dislodging it.
> - Regulate the drip rate of the secondary solution and adjust the rate of the primary solution.
> - Frequently monitor the patient and the infusion rate.
> - When the secondary infusion is finished, remove the needleless device from the injection port. Adjust the flow rate of the primary solution.

PATIENT-CONTROLLED ANALGESIA

PCA therapy allows your patient to control I.V. delivery of an analgesic (usually morphine) and maintain a therapeutic drug level. The computer-controlled PCA pump delivers a drug through an I.V. administration set that's attached directly to the patient's I.V. line. The patient can then push a button to receive a dose of analgesic through the I.V. line. Assess the patient regularly using the 0-to-10 scale for pain where 10 is the most severe pain. A timing unit prevents the patient from accidentally overdosing by imposing a lockout time between doses — usually 6 to 10 minutes. During this interval, the patient won't receive any analgesic despite pushing the button.

PCA therapy is indicated for patients who require parenteral analgesia. It's commonly used by patients after surgery and those with chronic diseases, particularly patients with terminal cancer or sickle cell anemia.

> **DOCUMENTATION TIP**
>
> ## Documenting I.V. drug administration
>
> After you administer an I.V drug, be sure to document:
> - drug and dosage
> - access site
> - duration of administration
> - patient's response
> - your name.

To receive PCA therapy, a patient must:
- be mentally alert
- understand and comply with instructions and procedures
- have no history of an allergy to the analgesic.

Patients not eligible for therapy include those with:
- limited respiratory reserve
- a history of drug abuse or chronic sedative or tranquilizer use
- a psychiatric disorder.

Patients receiving PCA therapy use fewer opioids for pain relief than other patients. PCA therapy also provides these advantages:
- It eliminates the need for I.M. analgesics.
- It provides individualized pain relief; each patient receives the correct dosage for his size and pain tolerance.
- It gives the patient a sense of control over pain.
- It allows the patient to sleep at night while minimizing daytime drowsiness.

The main adverse effect of opioid analgesics is respiratory depression. Therefore, you must routinely monitor your patient's respiratory rate. In addition to the effects on the respiratory system, opioid analgesics can lower blood pressure. If the opioid analgesic makes the patient nauseated, he may need an antiemetic.

When a patient is receiving PCA therapy be sure to check for infiltration into subcutaneous tissue and catheter occlusion, which may cause the drug to back up in the primary I.V. tubing.

The prescriber's order for PCA may include the:
- loading dose, which is given by bolus and is programmed by the infusion device
- lock-out interval, during which the PCA device can't be activated (such as every 6 to 10 minutes)
- maintenance dose, if a continuous infusion of opioid analgesia is ordered

- amount the patient will receive when the device is activated (such as 10 mg meperidine or 1 mg morphine)
- maximum amount the patient can receive within a specified time (usually the amount the patient can receive on demand or the maintenance dose over 60 minutes.)

Evaluating a PCA pump

In evaluating a PCA pump, first consider its cost and the cost of its operation. Ask yourself these questions:
- Does the pump use expensive refill cassettes or less expensive syringes?
- Consider the pump's complexity. How easy is it to operate — for you and the patient?
- What kind of lock-out mechanism is employed by the device? Operating the pump should be a straightforward procedure but not so simple that anyone can manipulate the program.
- Can the pump be used on an I.V pole and be carried or worn as well? Evaluate the equipment size and portability. An ambulatory patient should have a small, portable PCA pump.

PCA pumps are available with a variety of features:
- both continuous infusion and bolus doses or only bolus doses
- a wide range of volume settings
- a panel that displays the amount delivered or, if necessary, an alarm message
- can be programmed to record the concentration in either milligrams (mg) or milliliters (ml), allowing greater flexibility in choosing rates
- variable length of the lock-out interval from 5 to 90 minutes
- can be programmed to store and retrieve information such as the total dose allowed in a specified length of time
- can report the total volume infused to include the opioid analgesia in intake and output measurements.

Managing PCA therapy

With PCA, the patient self-administers the drug by pressing a button on a handheld controller that's connected to the pump. Before the device can be used it must be programmed to deliver specified doses at specified time intervals.

If the patient is using a pump that provides continuous infusion and bolus doses, make sure that he understands that he's receiving a drug continuously, but that he can give himself intermittent bolus doses for incidental pain (from coughing, for example) using the patient-control button.

If you program the pump to deliver a continuous infusion plus bolus doses, remember this rule: The cumulative doses per hour given by PCA shouldn't exceed the total hourly dose ordered by the prescriber. For example, if the patient needs a total of 6 mg of morphine over 1 hour, the prescriber may begin therapy with a continuous infusion of 3 mg/hour, allowing a bolus dose of 0.5 mg every 10 minutes.

A PCA pump that provides continuous infusion in addition to bolus doses will provide analgesia regardless of whether the patient uses the control button. This type of PCA is useful for helping patients cope with steady pain that gradually increases or decreases, incidental pain, or pain that's worse at different times. If the patient's pain is intermittent, he may not need continuous infusion.

Before allowing the patient to self-administer opioid analgesics with a PCA pump, his drug regimen should be reviewed. Simultaneous use of two central nervous system (CNS) depressants may cause drowsiness, oversedation, disorientation, and anxiety.

Explain to the patient how often he can self-administer the drug for pain. Reassure him that the lock-out interval will prevent him from giving the drug too frequently.

The prescriber may determine the initial trial bolus dose and time interval between boluses, according to the patient's condition and activity level. The prescriber orders ranges of dosing. The prescribed ranges are entered into the PCA pump's program. Once safe limits are set, the patient can push the button to receive a dose when he experiences pain. Reinforce how the PCA device works.

The prescriber may decide to change either the dose or the lock-out interval after close monitoring and thorough assessment of the patient.

These guidelines for determining an appropriate lock-out interval apply to both pumps that provide bolus doses only and pumps that provide bolus doses plus continuous infusions:

- For I.V. boluses, set the lock-out interval as prescribed by the prescriber. Typically, pain relief after an I.V. opioid bolus takes 6 to 10 minutes.
- For subQ boluses, set the lock-out interval for 30 minutes or more. Typically, pain relief after a subQ bolus takes 30 to 60 minutes.
- For spinal boluses, set the lock-out interval for 60 minutes or more. Typically pain relief after a spinal bolus takes 30 to 60 minutes.

If the patient isn't already receiving opioids, the pump is first programmed to deliver the drug until his pain is relieved (the loading dose). Then, the pump's hourly infusion rate is set to equal the total number of milligrams per hour. Check the patient's response every 15 to 30 minutes for 1 to 2 hours.

During therapy, monitor and record:
- amount of analgesic infused
- patient's respiratory rate
- patient's assessment of pain relief, using the 0-to-10 scale for pain where 10 is the most severe
- patient's level of consciousness.

If the patient doesn't feel that pain has been sufficiently relieved, notify the prescriber; he may increase the dosage.

Remember to monitor vital signs, especially when first starting therapy. Encourage the patient to practice coughing and deep breathing. This promotes ventilation and prevents pooling of secretions, which could lead to respiratory difficulty.

PCA complications

The primary complication of PCA administration is respiratory depression. If the patient's respiratory rate declines to 10 or fewer breaths per minute, call his name, touch him, and have him breathe deeply. If he's confused or restless or he can't be roused, stop the infusion, notify the prescriber, and give oxygen. Give an opioid antagonist such as naloxone.

Infiltration into subcutaneous tissue and catheter occlusion may also occur in PCA therapy as well as these complications:
- anaphylaxis
- nausea
- vomiting
- constipation
- orthostatic hypotension
- drug tolerance.

If prescribed, give the patient who experiences nausea an antiemetic such as chlorpromazine. If the patient has persistent nausea and vomiting during therapy the prescriber may change the drug.

Reinforce patient teaching

Make sure the patient and caregiver fully understand:
- how the pump works
- when to contact the prescriber
- signs and symptoms of adverse reactions
- signs and symptoms of drug tolerance.

Reinforce that the patient will be able to control his pain and that the pump is safe and effective. Remind him that an opioid analgesic relieves pain best when it's taken before the pain becomes intense. The patient should notify the prescriber if he fails to achieve adequate pain relief. The patient's caregiver should report signs of overdose: slow or irregular breathing, pinpoint pupils, and loss of consciousness. Teach the caregiver how to maintain respiration until help arrives.

Because an opioid analgesic may cause orthostatic hypotension, tell the patient to get up slowly from his bed or a chair. Instruct him to eat a high-fiber diet, drink plenty of fluids, and take a stool softener, if one has been prescribed. Caution him against drinking alcohol because this may enhance CNS depression.

Evaluate the effectiveness of the drug at regular intervals. Ask these questions:
- Is the patient getting relief?
- Does the dosage need to be increased because of persistent or worsening pain?
- Is the patient developing a tolerance to the drug?
- Is the patient's condition stable?

CHILDREN

Neonates and infants have precise fluid requirements. Keep in mind these considerations when you give I.V. drugs to children:
- Small children can't tolerate the large amount of fluid recommended for diluting many drugs.
- Because the drug dosage is based on the child's weight, each patient has a different normal dosing.
- Because of the small drug volume and slow delivery, you must make sure that no drug remains in the I.V. tubing before you change it.

Intermittent infusion

The most common method of giving I.V. drugs to children is by intermittent infusion, using a volume-control set.

When setting up the equipment for a child, take steps to ensure safety:
- Keep flow-control clamps out of the child's reach.
- Use tamper-proof pumps so the child can't change the rate inadvertently.
- Use an infusion pump with an anti-free-flow device that prevents inadvertent bolus infusions if the pump door is accidentally opened.

In many cases a child's venipuncture device must stay in place longer than an adult's. Protect the I.V. site from accidental dislodgment or contamination. Use sterile technique whenever you're giving I.V. drugs.

Retrograde administration

Retrograde administration offers one method for dealing with an infant's precise fluid requirements. This method uses coiled, low-volume tubing and a displacement syringe to prevent fluid overload.

ADVANTAGES

Retrograde administration allows an I.V. antibiotic to be administered over a 30-minute period without increasing the volume of fluid delivered to the patient. This method requires only one tubing to administer all I.V. fluids and drugs. The primary infusion rate doesn't have to be changed to administer I.V. drugs.

DISADVANTAGES

One downside of retrograde administration is that drug delivery is unpredictable, particularly with infusion rates of less than 5 ml/ hour. The low-volume tubing must be able to hold the entire diluted drug volume. If any is displaced into the syringe, it must be discarded.

The drug must be diluted in a volume equal to half that used at the milliliter-per-hour rate of the primary infusion; this allows for a 30-minute drug infusion. Therefore, if the primary rate is changed, the diluted drug volume must also be changed.

Syringe pump

A syringe pump is especially useful for giving intermittent I.V. drugs to children. It provides the greatest control for small-volume infusions. Make sure the pump is tamper-proof, has a built-in guard against uncontrolled infusion rates, and has an alarm sensitive to low-pressure occlusion. It should operate accurately with syringe sizes from 1 to 60 ml using low-volume tubing.

Intraosseous infusion

When venous access can't be established in an emergency, intraosseous infusion may be administered. This type of administration is the infusion of I.V. drug into a bone. Intraosseous infusion is usually performed by emergency personnel. It's a simple, quick, and relatively safe method for short-term emergency administration of lifesaving I.V. fluids and drugs.

Drugs used in intraosseous infusion may be given by continuous or intermittent infusion or by direct injection. Intraosseous infusion is as quick and effective as the I.V. route but should be used only until venous access can be established.

ELDERLY PATIENTS

When administering an I.V. analgesic to an elderly patient, watch closely for signs of respiratory or CNS depression such as confusion. When giving a drug that can cause renal toxicity, monitor the patient. Remember, the aging process alone means many elderly patients have decreased functioning in several of their biological systems.

Because many elderly patients have fragile veins, they're prone to infiltration and phlebitis. Carefully assess the I.V. site for signs and symptoms of these complications. If necessary, restart the infusion before you give a drug I.V.

Many I.V. drugs are particularly irritating to fragile veins, so you may have to dilute a drug in a larger volume than you normally would. Elderly patients are prone to fluid overload; keep accurate intake and output records, and include all fluids given for I.V. drug administration.

Managing complications

To protect a patient receiving I.V. therapy, watch for signs and symptoms of these serious complications:
- hypersensitivity
- extravasation
- infiltration
- phlebitis
- infection. (See *Managing complications of I.V. drug therapy,* pages 186 and 187.)

HYPERSENSITIVITY

Before you administer a drug, take steps to find out if your patient may be prone to hypersensitivity:
- Ask the patient if he has allergies, including ones to food or pollen.
- Ask if he has a family history of allergies. Patients with a personal or family history of allergies are more likely to develop a drug hypersensitivity.
- If your patient is an infant younger than age 3 months, be sure to ask the mother about her allergy history because maternal antibodies may still be present.

After giving an I.V. drug, follow through with these precautions:
- Stay with the patient for 5 to 10 minutes to detect early signs and symptoms of hypersensitivity, such as sudden fever, joint swelling, rash, urticaria, bronchospasm, and wheezing.

Managing complications of I.V. drug therapy

Use this table to correct possible complications of I.V. drug administration.

COMPLICATIONS	SIGNS AND SYMPTOMS	PURPOSE
Circulatory overload	• Neck vein distention or engorgement • Respiratory distress • Increased blood pressure • Crackles • Positive fluid balance	• Stop the infusion and place the patient in semi-Fowler's position, as tolerated. • Reduce the patient's anxiety. • Administer oxygen. • Notify the physician. • Administer diuretics. • Monitor the patient's vital signs
Hypersensitivity	• Itching, urticarial rash • Tearing eyes, runny nose • Bronchospasm • Wheezing • Anaphylactic reaction	• Stop the infusion. • Maintain a patent airway. • Administer an antihistaminic steroid, an anti-inflammatory drug, and an antipyretic. • Give 0.2 to 0.5 ml of 1:1,000 aqueous epinephrine subQ.; repeat at 3-minute intervals and as needed. • Monitor the patient's vital signs.
Infiltration (peripheral I.V.)	• Swelling • Discomfort • Burning • Tightness • Cool skin • Blanching	• Stop the infusion and remove the device (unless drug is a vesicant; in such cases, consult the pharmacy). • Elevate the limb. • Check the patient's pulse and capillary refill. • Restart the I.V. and infusion. • Document the patient's condition and interventions. • Check the site frequently.

■ If the patient is receiving a drug for the first time, check him every 5 to 10 minutes or according to your facility's policy. Otherwise check every 30 minutes for a few hours.

Managing complications of I.V. drug therapy
(*continued*)

COMPLICATIONS	SIGNS AND SYMPTOMS	PURPOSE
Phlebitis (peripheral I.V.)	• Redness or tenderness at the tip of the device • Puffy area over the vein • Elevated temperature	• Stop the infusion and remove the device. • Apply a warm pack. • Document the patient's condition and interventions. • Insert a new I.V. catheter using a larger vein or a smaller device and restart the infusion.
Systemic infection	• Elevated temperature • Malaise	• Stop the infusion. • Notify the physician. • Remove the device. • Culture the site and device as ordered. • Administer medications as prescribed. • Monitor the patient's vital signs.
Venous spasm	• Pain along the vein • Sluggish flow rate when clamp is completely open • Blanched skin over the vein	• Apply warm soaks over the vein and surrounding tissue. • Slow the flow rate.
Speed shock	• Headache • Syncope • Flushed face • Tightness in chest • Irregular pulse • Shock • Cardiac arrest	• Stop the infusion. • Call the physician. • Give dextrose 5% in water at keep-vein-open rate.

At the first sign of hypersensitivity, stop the infusion and notify the prescriber immediately. Immediate severe reactions are life-threatening. If necessary, assist with emergency treatment or resuscitation.

INFILTRATION

Infiltration commonly stems from improper placement or dislodgment of the catheter. In elderly patients, this complication may occur because the veins are thin and fragile.

The risk of infiltration increases when the tip is positioned near a flexion area. In this case, patient movement may cause the device to telescope within the vein or slip out or through the lumen of the vessel.

If only a small amount of an isotonic solution or nonirritating drug infiltrates, the patient usually experiences only mild discomfort. Routine comfort measures in this case include elevating the extremity. Document your infiltration findings using the infiltration scale. (See *The infiltration scale.*)

EXTRAVASATION

Extravasation, leaking of vesicant drugs such as various antineoplastic drugs and sympathomimetics, can produce severe local tissue damage, which may:
- cause discomfort
- delay healing
- produce infection and disfigurement
- lead to loss of function and possibly amputation.

For prevention tips, see *Preventing extravasation,* page 190.

If you suspect extravasation, follow your facility's protocol. Essential steps include the following:
- Stop the infusion and remove the I.V. line unless you need the catheter in place to instill the antidote.
- Estimate the amount of extravasated solution and notify the prescriber.
- Instill the appropriate antidote according to facility protocol.
- Elevate the extremity.
- Record the extravasation site, the patient's symptoms, the estimated amount of infiltrated solution, and the treatment. Record the time you notified the prescriber and his name. Continue documenting the appearance of the site and associated symptoms.
- Following manufacturer's recommendations, apply either ice packs or warm compresses to the affected area.

To determine if extravasation is occurring, nurses commonly test for blood return. But the absence of blood return doesn't always indicate extravasation, especially in these cases:
- You're using a small needle in a small vein or in one with low venous pressure

> **BEST PRACTICE**
>
> ## The infiltration scale
>
> The Intravenous Nurses Society Revised Standards of Practice have classified the degrees of infiltration. Use these classifications, outlined in the table below, when documenting instances of infiltration.
>
> | DEGREE | DESCRIPTION |
> |--------|-------------|
> | 0 | • No symptoms |
> | 1+ | • Skin blanched
• Edema less than 1" in any direction
• Cool to touch
• With or without pain |
> | 2+ | • Skin blanched
• Edema 1" to 6" in any direction
• Cool to touch
• With or without pain |
> | 3+ | • Skin blanched, translucent
• Gross edema more than 6" in any direction
• Cool to touch
• Mild to moderate pain
• Possible numbness |
> | 4+ | • Skin blanched, translucent, tight, leaking, discolored, bruised, swollen
• Gross edema more than 6" in any direction
• Deep, pitting tissue edema
• Circulatory impairment
• Moderate to severe pain
• Infiltration of any amount of blood product, irritant, or vesicant |

- The tip of the venous access device is lodged against the vein wall.

  Here's the truth about other common misconceptions:
- Extravasation doesn't always cause a hard lump. When the needle tip is completely out of the vein wall, a lump may form. But if fluid leaks out of the vein slowly (as it may when the catheter tip partially punctures the vein wall), extravasation may produce only a flat, diffuse swelling.

Preventing extravasation

Extravasation – the leaking of vesicant (blistering) drugs or fluids into the surrounding tissue – can occur when a vein is punctured or when there's leakage around an I.V. site. If extravasation occurs, severe local tissue damage may result. To prevent extravasation when you're giving vesicants, adhere strictly to proper administration techniques and follow the guidelines described here.

SITE SELECTION, VENIPUNCTURE, AND INFUSION

When preparing the patient for drug administration, keep these guidelines in mind:
- Don't use an existing I.V. line unless its patency is assured. Perform a new venipuncture to ensure correct needle placement and vein patency.
- Select the site carefully. Use a distal vein that allows successive venipunctures. To avoid tendon and nerve damage from possible extravasation, avoid using the back of the hand. Avoid the wrist and fingers (which are hard to immobilize) and areas previously damaged or that have poor circulation.
- Probing for a vein may cause trauma. Stop and begin again at another site.
- Always start the infusion with dextrose 5% in water (D_5W) or normal saline solution.

CHECK IT OUT

Check for infiltration before giving the drug. Apply a tourniquet above the needle to occlude the vein, and see if the flow continues. If the flow stops, the solution isn't infiltrating. Alternatively, simply lower the I.V. container and watch for blood backflow. The latter method is less reliable because the needle may have punctured the opposite vein wall though still resting partially in the vein. Flush the needle to ensure patency. If swelling occurs at the I.V. site, the solution is infiltrating.

DURING AND AFTER ADMINISTRATION

When you're ready to administer the drugs, follow these guidelines:
- Give the drugs by slow I.V. push through a free-flowing I.V. line or by small-volume infusion (50 to 100 ml).
- Give vesicants last when multiple drugs are ordered. If possible, avoid using an infusion pump to administer vesicants. A pump will continue the infusion if infiltration occurs.
- During administration, observe the infusion site for erythema or infiltration. Tell your patient to report any burning, stinging, pain, or sensation of sudden "heat" at the site.
- Use a transparent semipermeable dressing to allow frequent inspection of the I.V. site.
- After drug administration, instill several milliliters of D_5W or normal saline solution to flush the drug from the vein and prevent drug leakage when the catheter is removed.

- The patient may not always experience coldness or discomfort with extravasation. He may feel cold if extravasation occurs during rapid administration of a drug but, he will rarely feel cold from extravasation during a slow infusion.

PHLEBITIS

Postinfusion phlebitis is a common complication of I.V. therapy. It's usually associated with the following types of drugs or solutions:
- acidic
- alkaline
- high osmolarity.

Contributing factors include:
- vein trauma during insertion
- using a vein that's too small
- using an infusion device that's too large
- prolonged use of the same I.V. site.

Phlebitis can follow any infusion — or even an injection of a single drug — but it's more common after continuous infusions. Typically, phlebitis develops 2 to 3 days after the vein is exposed to the drug or solution. Phlebitis develops more rapidly in remote veins than in the larger veins close to the heart.

Drugs given by direct injection generally don't cause phlebitis when administered at the correct dilution and rate. Phenytoin and diazepam, which are frequently given by direct injection, can produce phlebitis after one or more injections at the same I.V. site.

Phlebitis is likely to occur when piggybacking certain irritating I.V. drugs, such as:
- erythromycin
- tetracycline
- nafcillin sodium
- vancomycin
- amphotericin B.

Large doses of potassium chloride (40 mEq/L or more), amino acids, dextrose solutions (10% or more), and multivitamins can also cause phlebitis.

If the patient's condition can tolerate it, add 250 to 1,000 ml of diluent to irritating drugs to help reduce the risk of irritation. You still should change the I.V. site every 72 hours or more frequently if necessary. If peripheral access is limited, suggest the placement of a central line to reduce the number of needle sticks, especially for long-term therapy.

Phlebitis can also result from motion and pressure of the infusion device. Particles in drugs and I.V. solutions can produce phle-

> **BEST PRACTICE**
>
> ## Detecting and classifying phlebitis
>
> If you detect phlebitis early, it can be treated effectively. If undetected, however, phlebitis can cause local infection, severe discomfort, and even sepsis.
>
> Phlebitis develops in the following way. As platelets aggregate at the damage site, a clot begins to form and histamine, bradykinin, and serotonin are released. Increased blood flow to the injury site and clot formation at the vein wall cause redness, tenderness, and slight swelling.
>
> If you don't remove the infusion device at this stage, the vein wall becomes hard and tender and may develop a red streak 2″ to 6″ (5 to 15 cm) long. Left untreated phlebitis may produce exudate at the I.V. site, accompanied by an elevated white blood cell count and fever. It can also produce pain at the I.V. site but a lack of pain doesn't eliminate the possibility of phlebitis.
>
> ### HOW TO CLASSIFY IT
> According to the Intravenous Nurses Society Revised Standards of Practice, the degrees of phlebitis are classified as:
>
> 0 = no clinical symptoms
> 1+ = erythema with or without pain
> 2+ = erythema with pain, edema may or may not be present
> 3+ = erythema with pain, edema may or may not be present, streak formation, palpable cord
> 4+ = erythema with pain, edema may or may not be present, streak formation, palpable cord longer than 1″, purulent drainage.

bitis, but you can reduce this risk by using filter needles and in-line filters.

To help prevent phlebitis, the pharmacist can alter drug osmolarity and pH without affecting the primary drug. Take the following measures:
- Use proper venipuncture technique.
- Dilute the drug correctly.
- Monitor administration rate.
- Observe the I.V. site frequently.
- Change the infusion site regularly.

To detect phlebitis, inspect the I.V. site several times per day. Use a transparent semipermeable dressing so you can see the skin covering the end of the access device as well as the insertion site. (See *Detecting and classifying phlebitis*.)

If you suspect phlebitis, follow these steps:
- At the first sign of redness or tenderness, move the venipuncture device to another site, preferably on the opposite arm.

- To ease your patient's discomfort, apply warm packs, or soak the arm in warm water.

INFECTION

A patient receiving I.V. drug therapy may develop a local infection at the I.V. site. Monitor the patient for signs and symptoms of infection, such as extreme redness and discharge at the site.

Keep in mind that you're at risk for exposure to serious infection. If your patient has the hepatitis B virus, human immunodeficiency virus, or another blood-borne pathogen, it can be transmitted to you through poor technique or failure to use standard precautions.

To protect yourself, follow the precautions for handling blood and body fluids recommended by the Centers for Disease Control and Prevention. Remember to treat all patients as potentially infected and take appropriate precautions. If you administer I.V. drugs and solutions, you should receive the hepatitis B vaccine (if you don't already have hepatitis B antibodies).

5

TRANSFUSIONS

Understanding transfusion therapy

The circulatory system is the body's main mover of blood and its components. The bloodstream carries oxygen, nutrients, hormones, and other vital substances to all body tissues and organs. When illness or injury decreases the blood's volume, oxygen-carrying capacity, or vital components, the introduction of whole blood or blood components directly into the bloodstream, or *transfusion therapy,* may be the only solution.

Most states allow nurses with RN licenses (but not LPN or LVN licenses) to administer blood and blood components. In some states, nurses with LPN licenses may regulate transfusion infusion rates, observe patients for reactions, stop transfusions, and document procedures. Know your state's nurse practice act and have the proper training before performing a transfusion or transfusion-related procedure.

PURPOSE OF TRANSFUSION THERAPY

Transfusion therapy's main purposes are:
- to restore and to maintain blood volume
- to improve the blood's oxygen-carrying capacity
- to replace deficient blood components and improve coagulation.

The average adult body contains about 5 L of blood. However, hemorrhage, trauma, or burns can send blood volume plunging. Restoring and maintaining blood volume is important because blood helps to maintain fluid balance. When blood transfusion is contraindicated in a patient, fluid infusions can restore circulatory volume. Unlike blood, fluid infusions can't improve oxygen-carrying capacity or replace deficient components.

When a person inhales, air surges into the lungs. Blood then harvests oxygen from the air mixture and carries it throughout the body. The blood's oxygen-carrying capacity may be depleted from

> **BEST PRACTICE**
>
> ## Protecting yourself from pathogens
>
> When caring for a patient who's receiving a blood transfusion, remember to protect yourself from exposure to transmissible diseases, such as viral hepatitis and human immunodeficiency virus. The Centers for Disease Control and Prevention guidelines recommend wearing gloves, a mask, goggles, and a gown when transfusing blood, in case of blood spills or sprays.

respiratory disorders, sepsis, carbon monoxide poisoning, pH imbalance, acute anemia from blood loss, sickle cell disease, or other chronic diseases. I.V. transfusion of red blood cell (RBC) components can help restore the role of blood in oxygen delivery.

The blood's coagulation capacity can be depleted by hemorrhage, liver failure, bone marrow suppression, platelet depletion (thrombocytopenia), drug- and disease-induced coagulopathies, or vitamin K deficiency. I.V. transfusion may be used to replace the blood's missing coagulation components.

METHODS OF TRANSFUSION THERAPY
Blood and blood products can be given in two ways: through a peripheral I.V. line or through a central venous (CV) line. Blood products can be transfused through a peripheral I.V. line, but it isn't the best idea if large volumes must be transfused quickly. It's recommended that an 18G or larger peripheral I.V. catheter be used for rapid transfusions in acute situations. Peripheral veins are frequently used in nonacute transfusion situations. The small diameter of the vein and peripheral resistance (resistance to blood flow in the vein) can slow the transfusion. Large volumes of blood products can be delivered quickly through a CV line because of the large size of the blood vessels and their decreased resistance to infusion.

RISKS IN TRANSFUSION THERAPY
Because of careful screening and testing, the blood supply is safer today than it has ever been. Even so, a patient who receives a transfusion is still at risk for life-threatening complications, such as a hemolytic reaction (which destroys RBCs), and exposure to infectious diseases, such as human immunodeficiency virus, and hepatitis. The physician, nurse, and patient (when able) must weigh the benefits of a transfusion against the risks. Patients must be informed of the risks of transfusions. Many facilities have special consent forms for transfusions. (See *Protecting yourself from pathogens*.)

Blood composition

Blood contains two basic components: cellular elements and plasma. Cellular elements, which make up about 45% of blood volume, include:
- erythrocytes, or red blood cells (RBCs)
- leukocytes, or white blood cells (WBCs)
- thrombocytes (platelets).

Plasma, the liquid component of blood, makes up about 55% of blood volume. The most significant components of plasma are water (serum) and protein (albumin, globulin, and fibrinogen). Other elements in plasma include:
- bilirubin
- carbohydrates
- electrolytes
- gases
- lipids
- nonprotein nitrogen compounds
- vitamins.

SEPARATING BLOOD FOR TRANSFUSION

Generally, only a patient who has lost a massive amount of blood in a short time requires a whole-blood transfusion. Most patients can be treated with individual *blood products* — the separate components that make up whole blood.

Current technology allows freshly donated whole blood to be separated into its component parts:
- RBCs
- plasma
- platelets
- leukocytes
- plasma proteins, such as immune globulin, albumin, and clotting factors.

Individual blood components can be used to correct specific blood deficiencies. The availability of blood components usually makes it unnecessary to transfuse whole blood.

TRANSFUSING CELLULAR PRODUCTS

The patient's condition dictates which type of cellular product is needed in transfusion therapy. (See *Guide to whole blood and cellular products,* pages 198 to 201.)

Commonly transfused cellular products include:
- whole blood

- packed RBCs
- leukocyte-poor RBCs
- WBCs
- platelets.

Whole blood and packed red blood cells
To replenish decreased blood volume or to boost the oxygen-carrying capacity of blood, the physician orders a transfusion of either whole blood or packed RBCs. If the patient is receiving whole blood or packed RBCs (blood from which 80% of the plasma has been removed), the blood shouldn't be obtained until just before the equipment is gathered because RBCs deteriorate after 4 hours at room temperature.

Whole blood transfusions are used to increase blood volume. They're usually needed because of massive hemorrhage (loss of more than 25% of total blood) resulting from trauma or vascular or cardiac surgery. Packed RBCs are transfused to maintain or restore oxygen-carrying capability. They can also replace RBCs lost because of a GI bleed, dysmenorrhea, surgery, trauma, or chemotherapy.

Leukocyte-poor red blood cells
Leukocyte-poor RBCs are transfused when a patient has had a febrile, nonhemolytic transfusion reaction, caused by WBC antigens reacting with the patient's WBC antibodies or platelets. Several methods are used to remove leukocytes from blood:
- centrifugal force along with filtration and the addition of sedimentary agents, such as dextran and hydroxyethyl starch
- leukocyte removal filters
- washing the cells in a special solution (the most expensive and the least effective method; it also removes about 99% of the plasma).

White blood cells
Transfusion of granulocytes (leukocytes containing granules) may be ordered to fight antibiotic-resistant septicemia and other life-threatening infections or when granulocyte supply is severely low (granulocytopenia). This therapy is repeated for 4 to 5 days or longer, as ordered, unless the bone marrow recovers or severe reactions occur. Because some RBCs normally remain in WBC concentrates, granulocytes are tested for compatibility (ABO, Rh, and human leukocyte antigen).

(Text continues on page 200.)

Guide to whole blood and cellular products

BLOOD COMPONENT AND VOLUME | INDICATIONS

WHOLE BLOOD
Complete (pure) blood
Volume: 500 ml

- To restore blood volume in hemorrhaging, trauma, or burn patients

PACKED RED BLOOD CELLS (RBCs)
Same RBC mass as whole blood with 80% of the plasma removed
Volume: 250 ml

- To restore or maintain oxygen-carrying capacity
- To correct anemia and surgical blood loss
- To increase RBC mass

LEUKOCYTE-POOR RBCs
Same as packed RBCs except 70% of the leukocytes are removed
Volume: 200 ml

- To restore or maintain oxygen-carrying capacity
- To correct anemia and surgical blood loss
- To increase RBC mass
- To prevent febrile reactions from leukocyte antibodies
- To treat immunosuppressed patients
- To restore RBCs to patients who have had two or more nonhemolytic febrile reactions

Nursing considerations

- Compatability is ABO identical.
- Group A receives A; group B receives B; group AB receives AB; group O receives O. Rh type must match.
- Use blood administration tubing; can infuse rapidly in emergencies, but adjust the rate to the patient's condition and the transfusion order, and don't infuse over more than 4 hours.
- Whole blood is seldom administered other than in emergency situations because its components can be extracted and administered separately.

- Compatability: Group A receives A or O; group B receives B or O; group AB receives AB, A, B, or O; group O receives O. Rh type must match.
- Use blood administration tubing; can infuse rapidly in emergencies. The rate is adjusted to the patient's condition and the transfusion order, and the infusion shouldn't be over more than 4 hours.
- RBCs have the same oxygen-carrying capacity as whole blood, minimizing the hazard of volume overload.
- Using packed RBCs avoids potassium and ammonia buildup that sometimes occurs in the plasma of stored blood.
- Packed RBCs shouldn't be used for anemic conditions correctable by nutrition or drug therapy.

- Compatibility: Group A receives A or O; group B receives B or O; group AB receives AB, A, B, or O; group O receives O. Rh type must match.
- Use blood administration tubing. May require a microaggregate filter (40-micron filter) for hard-spun, leukocyte-poor RBCs. Infuse over 1 1/2 to 4 hours.
- Cells expire 24 hours after washing.
- RBCs have the same oxygen-carrying capacity as whole blood, minimizing the hazard of volume overload.
- Leukocyte-poor RBCs shouldn't be used for anemic conditions correctable by nutrition or drug therapy.

(continued)

Guide to whole blood and cellular products (*continued*)

BLOOD COMPONENT AND VOLUME	INDICATIONS
WHITE BLOOD CELLS (WBCs, LEUKOCYTES) Whole blood with all the RBCs and 80% of the plasma removed Volume: 150 ml	• To treat life-threatening granulocytopenia (granulocyte count less than 500/µl) in a patient who isn't responding to antibiotics, especially if he has positive blood cultures or a persistent fever greater than 101° F (38.3° C)
PLATELETS Platelet sediment from RBCs or plasma Volume: 35 to 50 ml/unit; 1 unit of platelets=7 x 10^7 platelets	• To treat thrombocytopenia caused by decreased platelet production, increased platelet destruction, or massive transfusion of stored blood • To treat acute leukemia and marrow aplasia • To restore platelet count in a preoperative patient with a count of 100,000/µl or less

Platelets

Platelets can be transfused to control or prevent bleeding or correct an extremely low platelet count (20,000/µl or less) in a patient who doesn't have a disease that destroys platelets. They're also transfused to increase the number of platelets in a patient who's receiving a platelet-destroying therapy, such as chemotherapy, or who has a hematologic disease, such as aplastic anemia or leukemia.

Nursing considerations

- Compatibility: Group A receives A or O; group B receives B or O; group AB receives AB, A, B, or O; group O receives O. Rh type must match. WBCs are preferably human leukocyte antigen (HLA)-compatible, but not necessary unless patient is HLA-sensitized from previous transfusions.
- Use blood administration tubing. One unit daily is given for 4 to 6 days or until infection clears.
- WBC infusion may induce fever and chills. To prevent this reaction, the patient is premedicated with antihistamines, acetaminophen (Tylenol), steroids, or meperidine (Demerol). If fever occurs, give an antipyretic, but don't stop the transfusion. Reduce the flow rate for the patient's comfort.
- Because reactions are common, administer slowly over 2 to 4 hours. Check the patient's vital signs and assess him every 15 minutes throughout the transfusion.
- Give the transfusion with antibiotics to treat infection.

- Compatibility: ABO identical when possible. Rh negative recipients should receive Rh negative platelets when possible.
- Use a filtered blood component drip administration set; infuse 100 ml over 15 minutes. Administer at 150 to 200 ml/hour, or as rapidly as the patient can tolerate; don't exceed 4 hours. Don't use a microaggregate filter.
- Platelet transfusions aren't usually indicated for conditions of accelerated platelet destruction, such as idiopathic thrombocytopenic purpura or drug-induced thrombocytopenia.
- Patients with a history of platelet reaction require premedication with antipyretics and antihistamines. A leukocyte removal filter may be necessary.
- If the patient has a fever, don't give platelets.
- A blood platelet count may be ordered 1 hour after platelet transfusion to determine platelet transfusion increments.

Blood type compatibility

Recipient blood is choosy about donor blood. An incompatibility can cause serious adverse reactions. The most severe is a hemolytic reaction, which destroys red blood cells (RBCs) and may become life-threatening. Before a transfusion, testing helps to detect incompatibilities between recipient and donor blood.

Typing and crossmatching establish the compatibility of donor and recipient blood. This precaution minimizes the risk of a hemolytic reaction. The most important tests include:

- ABO blood typing
- Rh typing
- crossmatching
- direct antiglobulin test
- antibody screening test
- screening for such diseases as hepatitis B and C, human immunodeficiency virus, human T-cell lymphotrophic virus type I and type II (hairy cell leukemia), syphilis and, for certain patients, cytomegalovirus.

ABO BLOOD TYPE

The blood types in the ABO system are A, B, both of these (AB), or neither (O). Each blood type is named for a substance carried by the RBCs that can stimulate the formation of an antibody, or *antigen*. An antigen may induce the formation of a corresponding antibody if given to a person who doesn't normally carry the antigen.

An *antibody* is an immunoglobulin molecule synthesized in response to a specific antigen. The ABO system includes two naturally occurring antibodies: anti-A and anti-B. One, both, or neither of these antibodies may be found in the plasma. The interaction of corresponding antigens and antibodies of the ABO system can cause agglutination (clumping together).

The major antigens, such as those in the ABO system, are inherited. Blood transfusions can introduce other antigens and antibodies into the body. Most are harmless, but any could cause a transfusion reaction.

A hemolytic reaction occurs when donor and recipient blood types are mismatched. This could happen, for example, if blood containing anti-A antibodies is transfused to a recipient who has blood with A antigens. (See *Blood type compatibility*.)

RED FLAG *A hemolytic reaction can be life-threatening. With as little as 10 ml infused, symptoms can occur quickly — including headache, chest pain, chills, back pain, and fever. Because this reaction is so fast, always adhere strictly to your facility's policy and procedures for assessing the patient's vital signs during transfusions.*

When mismatching occurs, antigens and antibodies of the ABO system do battle. Antibodies attach to the surfaces of the recipient's RBCs, causing the cells to clump together (agglutinate). Eventually, the clumped cells can plug small blood vessels. This antibody-antigen reaction activates the body's complement system, a group of enzymatic proteins that cause RBC destruction (hemolysis). RBC hemolysis releases free hemoglobin (an RBC component) into the

Blood type compatibility

Precise typing and crossmatching of donor and recipient blood helps avoid transfusing incompatible blood, which can be fatal. This chart shows ABO compatibility for the recipient and donor.

Blood Type	**Antibodies in Plasma**	**Compatible Red Blood Cells**	**Compatible Plasma**
Recipient			
O	Anti-A and anti-B	O	O, A, B, AB
A	Anti-B	A, O	A, AB
B	Anti-A	B, O	B, AB
AB	Neither anti-A nor anti-B	AB, A, B, O	AB
Donor			
O	Anti-A and anti-B	O, A, B, AB	O
A	Anti-B	A, AB	A, O
B	Anti-A	B, AB	B, O
AB	Neither anti-A nor anti-B	AB	AB, A, B, O

bloodstream, which can damage renal tubules and lead to kidney failure.

Because type O blood lacks A and B antigens, it can be transfused in limited amounts in an emergency to any patient — regardless of the recipient's blood type — with little risk of adverse reaction. That's why the patient with type O blood is called a *universal donor*.

A patient with AB blood type has neither anti-A nor anti-B antibodies. This patient may receive A, B, AB, or O blood, making him a *universal recipient*.

RH BLOOD TYPE

Another major blood antigen system, the Rhesus (Rh) system, has two blood types: Rh-positive and Rh-negative. The Rh system consists of different inherited antigens—D, C, E, c, or e. These antigens are highly immunogenic—they have a high capacity for initiating the body's immune response. D, or D factor, is the most important Rh antigen. The presence or absence of D is one of the factors that determine whether a person has Rh-positive or Rh-negative blood.

Rh-positive blood contains a variant of the D antigen or D factor; Rh-negative blood doesn't have this antigen. A person with Rh-negative blood who receives Rh-positive blood will gradually develop anti-Rh antibodies. The first exposure won't cause a reaction because anti-Rh antibodies are slow to form. Subsequent exposures, however, may pose a risk of hemolysis and agglutination. Some other unique characteristics of the Rh blood type for you to think about:

- A patient with Rh-positive blood doesn't carry anti-Rh antibodies because they would destroy his own RBCs.
- Nearly 95% of Blacks, Native Americans, and Asians have Rh-positive blood; about 85% of Whites have Rh-positive blood. The rest of the population has Rh-negative blood.
- There are two ways Rh-positive blood can get into Rh-negative blood: by transfusion or during a pregnancy in which the fetus has Rh-positive blood. (See *Managing an Rh pregnancy*.)

HUMAN LEUKOCYTE ANTIGENS

Human leukocyte antigens (HLAs) are essential to immunity. HLA is part of the histocompatibility system. This system controls compatibility between transplant or transfusion recipients and donors. The HLA system:

- is responsible for graft success or rejection (Generally, the closer the HLA match between donor and recipient, the less likely the tissue or organ will be rejected.)
- may be involved with host defense against cancer
- may be involved when white blood cells (WBCs) or platelets fail to multiply after being transfused (if this happens, the HLA system could trigger a fatal immune reaction in the patient).

HLA testing benefits patients receiving massive, multiple, or frequent transfusions. HLA evaluation is also conducted for patients who:

- will receive platelet and WBC transfusions
- will undergo organ or tissue transplantation
- have severe or refractory febrile transfusion reactions.

> **BEST PRACTICE**
>
> ## Managing an Rh pregnancy
>
> Rh factor incompatibility can cause a problem in pregnancy if a mother has Rh-negative blood and her fetus inherits Rh-positive blood from the father. During her first pregnancy, the woman becomes sensitized to Rh-positive fetal blood factors, but her antibodies usually aren't sufficient to harm the fetus. Sensitization may occur after a miscarriage or an abortion.
>
> In a subsequent pregnancy with an Rh-positive fetus, increasing amounts of the mother's anti-Rh antibodies attack the fetus, destroying red blood cells (RBCs). As the fetus's body produces new RBCs, cell destruction escalates, releasing bilirubin (a red cell component). The fetal liver's inability to properly process and excrete bilirubin can cause jaundice (soon after birth), other liver problems and possibly brain damage
>
> A severely affected infant may develop life-threatening hemolytic disease. Giving Rh immune globulin (RhoGAM) by I.M. injection within 72 hours after delivery or termination of pregnancy prevents the formation of anti-Rh antibodies, preventing the development of hemolytic disease in the neonate.

Giving transfusions

There are two kinds of transfused blood: autologous (from the recipient himself) and homologous (from a donor). Autologous blood reduces the risks normally associated with transfusions, but it may not be available. Homologous blood undergoes rigorous screening and testing to ensure its quality. Part of this screening involves the donors themselves. (See *Who can and can't donate blood, page 206.*)

The main concern during blood administration is to prevent a potentially fatal hemolytic reaction by making sure that the patient receives the correct product. You can help by making sure these steps are followed:

- An informed consent form should be signed.
- The patient's name, medical record number, ABO and Rh status (and other compatibility factors), and blood bank identification number should be checked against the label on the blood bag.
- The expiration date on the bag should be checked.
- All information should be verified by another nurse or physician according to facility policy. (Some facilities routinely require double identification.)

Who can and can't donate blood

Donors must be screened to reduce the risks associated with transfusions.

ELIGIBLE DONORS
- At least age 17 (age 16 in some states)
- Weigh at least 110 lb (50 kg)
- Must be healthy
- Not have donated in the past 56 days
- Hemoglobin level of at least 12.5 g/dl for women or 13.5 g/dl for men and hematocrit of at least 38%

INELIGIBLE
- Human immunodeficiency virus or acquired immunodeficiency syndrome
- Taken money or other payment for sex since 1977
- Man who has had sex with other men since 1977
- Taken illegal I.V. drugs
- Sex with prostitutes in the past 12 months
- Sex with anyone in the above categories in the past 12 months
- Hepatitis caused by a virus since age 11 or exposure in the past 12 months
- Certain types of cancer (not minor skin cancer)
- Bleeding conditions
- Received clotting factor concentrates
- Treated for syphilis or gonorrhea in the past 12 months
- Tattooed within the past 12 months
- Fever, infection, cold, or flu
- For donors with high blood pressure, systolic blood pressure less than 180 and diastolic less than 100
- Received a blood transfusion in the United States in the past 12 months or a transfusion in the United Kingdom (UK), Gibraltar, or Falkland Islands since 1980
- Received a blood transfusion in certain African countries since 1977
- Received a dura mater transplant or human pituitary growth hormone
- A blood relative with Creutzfeldt-Jacob disease
- Received bovine insulin made from cattle in the UK since 1980
- Hereditary hemochromatosis
- Were born or lived in Cameroon, Central African Republic, Chad, Congo, Equatorial Guinea, Gabon, Niger, or Nigeria since 1977
- Received smallpox vaccine in the past 56 days
- Treated for malaria, lived in a country where malaria is found in the past 3 years, or visited such a country in the past year
- Kidney transplant in the past year
- Pregnant
- Sickle cell disease
- Tuberculosis

Donors taking isotretinoin (Accutane), dutasteride (Avodart), or warfarin (Coumadin) must wait a specified time before donating.

- The blood confirmation slip should be signed by the staff member giving the blood and the nurse or physician who checked the blood or blood product. If even a slight discrepancy exists, the blood or blood product shouldn't be given. Instead, make sure the blood bank is notified immediately and the blood or blood product is returned.
- The blood or blood product should be inspected to detect abnormalities, such as for abnormal color, clumping of red blood cells (RBCs), gas bubbles, and extraneous material that might indicate bacterial contamination. If any of these signs are present, the bag should be returned to the blood bank.
- The patient's identity should be confirmed by checking the name, room number, and bed number on his wristband and, if possible, with the patient himself.

SELECTING EQUIPMENT

Before a transfusion is started, the following equipment is gathered:
- gloves, a gown, a mask, and goggles to wear when handling blood products
- in-line or add-on filters as specified by the physician's order or as appropriate for the product being infused
- I.V. pole
- transfusion component, exactly as ordered
- venipuncture equipment, if necessary.

No I.V. solution other than normal saline should be given with blood. If a primary line has been used to deliver a solution other than normal saline, a blood administration set shouldn't be affixed, or piggybacked, to it without first flushing the line.

Blood filters should always be used on blood products to avoid infusing fibrin clots or cellular debris that forms in the blood bag. There are many types of filters, each with unique features and indications. A standard blood administration set comes with a 170-micron filter, which traps particles that are 170 microns or larger. This filter doesn't remove smaller particles, called *microaggregates*, which form after only a few days of blood storage.

Microaggregates form from degenerating platelets and fibrin strands and may contribute to the formation of small clots, or microemboli, that obstruct circulation in the lungs. To remove microaggregates, the physician may order a 20- to 40-micron filter, called a *microaggregate filter.* This filter removes smaller particles but is costly and may slow the infusion rate—a particular problem when seeking to deliver a massive, rapid transfusion.

Filters may be used to screen out leukocytes during the transfusion of RBCs or platelets. Use new tubing and a new filter for every

1 to 2 units of blood that's transfused. A microaggregate filter should never be used to transfuse white blood cell concentrates or platelets; the filter will trap them. Instead, a leukocyte reduction filter specific for the component should be used.

A blood warmer may be ordered:
- to prevent hypothermia (for example, from large volumes of blood administered quickly)
- to prevent arrhythmias from hypothermia (86° F [30° C])
- when antibodies called *cold agglutinins* are present because they react at temperatures below 68° F (20° C) and can cause agglutination of the blood.

In some facilities, an infusion pump is used to regulate the administration of blood and blood products. The manufacturer's instructions should be checked to find out whether a particular pump can be used to administer blood or blood products.

STARTING THE TRANSFUSION

So far, you have identified the patient, inspected and verified the blood product and obtained the patient's baseline vital signs. If your state nurse practice act and facility policy allow, you may assemble and prepare the necessary equipment and supplies. Now the transfusion can be started. (See *Starting a transfusion*.)

After the transfusion has been started, the patient should be assessed and his vital signs monitored according to the patient's transfusion history and your facility's policy — usually every 15 minutes for the first hour.

MONITORING THE TRANSFUSION

To help avoid transfusion reactions and safeguard the patient, make sure these guidelines are followed:
- The patient's vital signs should be recorded before the transfusion, 15 minutes after the start of the transfusion, and just after the transfusion is complete, and more frequently if warranted by the patient's condition and transfusion history or the facility's policy. Most acute hemolytic reactions occur during the first 30 minutes of the transfusion, so the patient should be watched carefully during the first 30 minutes.
- Sterile normal saline solution, an isotonic solution, should always be set up as a primary line along with the transfusion.
- If the patient develops wheezing and bronchospasm, prompt action should be taken. These signs may indicate an allergic reaction or anaphylaxis. If, after a few milliliters of blood are transfused, the patient becomes dyspneic and shows generalized flushing and chest pain (with or without vomiting and diarrhea),

Starting a transfusion

If your state nurse practice act and facility policy allow, you may assist with this procedure. To transfuse, these steps should be followed.

LET'S BEGIN
- The procedure should be explained to the patient and consent obtained according to facility policy.
- Hands should be washed and gloves, a gown, goggles, and a mask donned.
- If a straight-line set is used, the set's tubing spike should be inserted into the bag of normal saline solution.
- The bag should be hung on the I.V. pole and the filter and tubing primed with saline solution to reduce the risk of microclots forming in the tubing. The bag of normal saline solution should be left attached to the tubing until the transfusion starts.

READY TO START
- A Y-type blood administration set should be used. Blood and saline are both connected and can be clamped without opening the system.
- The clamp should be removed from the normal saline solution line and the spike inserted on the regular administration set into the bag of saline solution and prime the line.
- When a Y-type set is used, all the clamps on the set should be closed. Then the spike of the line you're using for the normal saline solution should be inserted into the bag of normal saline solution. Next, the port

HANGING THE BAG

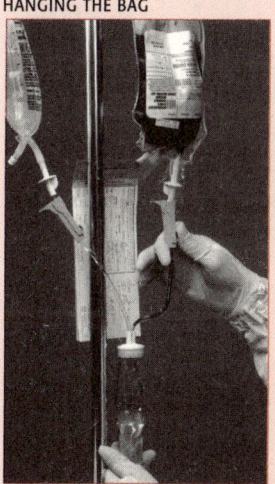

ADJUSTING THE CLAMP

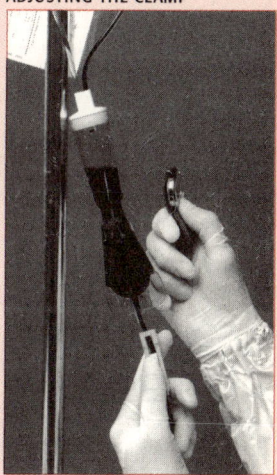

Starting a transfusion (continued)

on the blood bag should be opened and the spike of the line you're using to administer the blood or cellular component should be inserted into the port. The bag of normal saline solution and blood or cellular component should be hung on the I.V. pole, as shown.

- The clamp on the line of normal saline solution should be opened, and the drip chamber squeezed until it's half full of normal saline solution. Then the adapter cover at the tip of the blood administration set should be removed, the main flow clamp opened, and the tubing primed with normal saline solution. The clamp should be closed and the adapter recapped.

THE TRANSFUSION ITSELF
To transfuse blood or a cellular component, these steps should be followed:

- The patient's vital signs should be taken to serve as baseline values. His vital signs should be rechecked after 15 minutes (or according to facility policy).
- If the patient doesn't have an I.V. device in place, a venipuncture should be done using a 20G or larger catheter.
- The prepared blood administration set should be attached to the venous access device using a needleless connection and flushed with normal saline solution.
- When a Y-type set is used, the clamp on the normal saline solution line should be opened and the main flow clamped.
- When whole blood or white blood cells are given, the bag should be gently inverted several times during the procedure to mix the cells. (During the transfusion, the bag should be gently agitated to prevent the viscous cells from settling.)
- After the infusion device is flushed, the transfusion is begun.
- The clamp closest to the patient is adjusted to deliver a slow rate (usually about 20 gtt/minute) for the first 10 to 30 minutes. The type of blood product given and the patient's condition determine the rate of transfusion. A unit of red blood cells (RBCs) may be given over a period of 1 to 4 hours; platelets and coagulation factors may be given more quickly than RBCs and granulocytes.
- A transfusion shouldn't take longer than 4 hours because the risk of contamination and sepsis increases after that. Any blood or blood products not given within this time should be discarded or returned to the blood bank, as facility policy directs.

---

he could be having an anaphylactic reaction. The transfusion should be stopped immediately, the normal saline solution started, the patient's vital signs checked and documented, the physician called, and anaphylaxis procedure started.

- If the patient develops a transfusion reaction, the remaining blood should be returned together with a posttransfusion blood sample and other required specimens to the blood bank.

Best practice

Transfusion don'ts

A transfusion requires extreme care. Here are some tips on what shouldn't be done when a transfusion is given:
- Drugs should never be added to the blood bag.
- Blood products should never be given without checking the order against the blood bag label – the only way to tell if the request form has been stamped with the wrong name. Most life-threatening reactions occur when this step is omitted.
- If a discrepancy in the blood number, blood slip type, or patient identification number is discovered, the blood product shouldn't be transfused.
- Blood shouldn't be piggybacked into the port of an existing infusion set. Most solutions, including dextrose in water, are incompatible with blood. Blood should only be given with normal saline solution.
- If the patient shows changes in vital signs, is dyspneic or restless, or develops chills, hematuria, or pain in the flank, chest, or back the transfusion should be stopped. He could go into shock, so the I.V. device that's in place shouldn't be removed. It should be kept open with a slow infusion of normal saline solution; the physician and the laboratory should be called.

Signs or symptoms of a transfusion reaction include:
- fever
- chills
- rigor
- headache
- nausea
- back or flank pain
- restlessness.

If any of these signs or symptoms are detected, the transfusion should be stopped quickly and the normal saline solution infusion reestablished. If a Y-set is used, the infusion shouldn't be restarted by opening the clamp; that will just deliver more of the blood that's causing the problem. Instead, a new bag and tubing should be used to restart the infusion.

Next, the patient's vital signs should be checked and recorded. The physician should be notified immediately without disposing of the blood. If no signs of a reaction appear within 15 minutes, the flow clamp can be adjusted to achieve the ordered infusion rate. The patient should be monitored throughout the entire transfusion according to your facility's policy and procedures. (See *Transfusion don'ts*.)

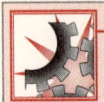

EQUIPMENT CHALLENGE

The pressure is on

Rapid blood replacement requires transfusing blood under pressure. Your state practice act and facility policy may not allow you to perform this procedure, however, it is important for you to understand how it is done. A pressure cuff is placed over the blood bag like a sleeve and inflated. The pressure gauge, attached to the cuff, is calibrated in millimeters of mercury (mm Hg). These steps should be followed when using blood under pressure:

- The patient is prepared and the equipment set up as with a straight-line blood administration set.
- The filter and tubing should be primed with normal saline solution to remove all air from the administration set.
- The tubing is connected to the needle or catheter hub.
- By increasing the pressure, the speed at which complications, such as infiltration, can occur also increases. The patient should be watched closely.
- A hand should be inserted into the top of the pressure cuff sleeve and the blood bag pulled up through the center opening. Then the blood bag loop is hung on the hook provided with the sleeve.
- The pressure cuff and blood bag is hung on the I.V. pole. The flow clamp on the tubing is opened.
- To set the flow rate, the screw clamp on the pressure cuff is turned counterclockwise. The pressure bulb of the cuff is compressed to inflate the bag until you achieve the desired flow rate. Then the screw clamp should be turned clockwise to maintain this constant flow rate.
- As the blood bag empties, the pressure decreases; the flow rate should be checked regularly and the pressure in the pressure cuff adjusted as necessary to maintain a consistent rate. The cuff needle shouldn't exceed 300 mm Hg; excessively high pressure can cause hemolysis and damage the component container or rupture the blood bag.

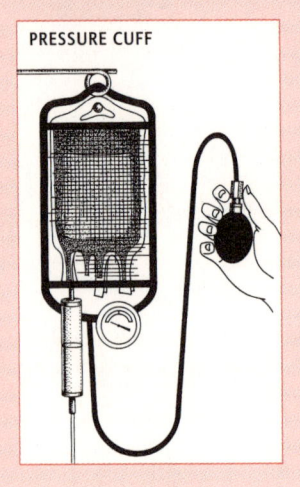

PRESSURE CUFF

> **DOCUMENTATION TIPS**
>
> ## Documenting blood transfusion
>
> Make sure that these items are recorded:
> - date and time of the transfusion
> - identification number on the blood bag
> - type and amount of blood transfused
> - volume of normal saline solution infused
> - status of the venous access device
> - patient's vital signs
> - signs or symptoms of a reaction (or the absence of signs or symptoms)
> - how the patient tolerated the procedure.

A pressure cuff on the blood container can increase the infusion rate. If one is used, make sure that it's equipped with a pressure gauge and that it exerts uniform compression against all parts of the container. The manufacturer's guidelines should be checked before using these devices for giving blood or blood components. (See *The pressure is on.*)

STOPPING THE TRANSFUSION

After a transfusion is complete, these steps should be followed:
- The blood tubing should be flushed with an adequate amount of normal saline solution according to the patient's condition.
- On a Y-type set, the clamp should be closed on the blood line and opened on the saline solution line.
- The tubing, filter, and blood bag should be discarded according to facility policy.
- The patient's condition and vital signs should be reassessed.
- The procedure should be documented. (See *Documenting blood transfusion.*)

Giving plasma and plasma fraction transfusions

Plasma and plasma fractions are the anticoagulated clear portion of blood that's been run through a centrifuge. They make up about 55% of blood and are used in transfusion therapy to:
- correct blood deficiencies such as a low platelet count

- control bleeding tendencies that result from clotting factor deficiencies
- increase the patient's circulating blood volume.

Before a transfusion, the plasma or plasma fractions are obtained. Commonly transfused plasma products include:
- fresh frozen plasma (FFP)
- albumin
- cryoprecipitate
- prothrombin complex.

The patient's condition dictates which plasma product is needed. (See *Guide to plasma products,* pages 216 and 217.)

Plasma substitutes may be used to maintain blood volume in an emergency, such as acute hemorrhage and shock. Plasma substitutes lack oxygen-carrying and coagulation properties, but using them allows time to get the patient's blood typed and crossmatched. Depending on the circumstances, a synthetic volume expander, such as dextran in saline solution, or a natural volume expander, such as plasma protein fraction and albumin, may be used.

SELECTING EQUIPMENT

The following equipment is needed:
- in-line or add-on filters or a filter system designated for the ordered component (usually a 170-micron filter) (Never use a microaggregate filter to infuse platelets or plasma; it could remove essential components from the transfusion.)
- normal saline solution
- I.V. pole
- clean gloves, a gown, a mask, and goggles
- ordered plasma or plasma fractions
- venipuncture equipment, if necessary.

STARTING THE TRANSFUSION

These steps are followed to begin the transfusion:
- The patient should have a functional venous access device (20G or greater).
- Clean gloves and other protective equipment that your facility requires should be donned.
- The blood product should be verified that it's correct and that it matches the number designated for the patient.
- The expiration date of the plasma or plasma fraction should be checked.
- Double-check that the right plasma or plasma fractions is being given.

> **DOCUMENTATION TIPS**
>
> ## Documenting transfusion of plasma or plasma products
>
> When plasma or plasma products have been infused, the following is recorded:
> - the type and amount of plasma or plasma fraction administered
> - duration of transfusion
> - the patient's baseline vital signs
> - adverse reactions
> - how the patient tolerated the procedure.

- The plasma or plasma fraction should be inspected for cloudiness and turbidity, which could indicate possible contamination.
- The bag should be spiked with component-specific tubing (if the blood bank provided it or with the blood tubing specified by your facility's policy and procedures).
- The tubing should be primed.
- The procedure should be explained to the patient.
- The patient's baseline vital signs should be obtained, and vital signs should be checked frequently according to your facility's policy.
- The patient's infusion device should be flushed with normal saline solution.
- The plasma, FFP, albumin, factor VIII concentrate, prothrombin complex, platelets, or cryoprecipitate should be attached to the patient's venous access device.
- The transfusion should be begun and adjusted to the ordered infusion rate.
- The patient's vital signs should be taken, and he should be assessed frequently for signs or symptoms of a transfusion reaction, such as fever, chills, or nausea. If a reaction occurs, the infusion should be quickly stopped and a normal saline solution infusion started at a keep-vein-open rate. The patient's vital signs should be checked and recorded. The physician should be notified.
- After the infusion, the line should be flushed with saline solution, according to facility policy. Then the I.V. line should be disconnected. If therapy will continue, the original I.V. solution should be hung and the flow rate adjusted.
- The procedure should be documented. (See *Documenting transfusion of plasma or plasma products*.)

(Text continues on page 222.)

Guide to plasma products

This table lists various plasma products and their indications for transfusion along with relevant nursing considerations for each.

BLOOD COMPONENT AND VOLUME	INDICATIONS
FRESH FROZEN PLASMA (FFP) Uncoagulated plasma separated from red blood cells. FFP is rich in coagulation factors V, VIII, and IX. Volume: 200 to 250 ml	• To correct an undetermined coagulation factor deficiency • Plasmapheresis replacement • To correct deficiencies • Hemorrhage • Warfarin reversal
ALBUMIN 5% (BUFFERED SALINE) ALBUMIN 25% (SALT-POOR) Human albumin is a small plasma protein separated from plasma. Volume: 5% = (50 mg/ml) in 50-ml, 250-ml, 500-ml, and 1,000-ml vials 25% = (250 mg/ml) in 20-ml, 50-ml, and 100-ml vials	• To replace volume in treatment of shock from burns, trauma, acute liver failure, or infections • To treat hypoproteinemia (with or without edema) • Pancreatitis • Neonatal hemolytic disease
FACTOR VIII (ANTIHEMOPHILIC FACTOR) Cold insoluble portion of plasma recovered from FFP Volume: specific to the product	• To treat a patient with hemophilia A with joint hemorrhages or other bleeding episodes • Preparation for elective or emergency surgery in patients with hemophilia A • Von Willebrand disease
FACTORS II, VII, IX, X COMPLEX (PROTHROMBIN COMPLEX) Lyophilized commercially prepared solution drawn from pooled plasma Volume: specific to the product	• To treat a congenital factor V deficiency and other bleeding disorders resulting from an acquired deficiency of factors II, VII, IX, and X

Giving plasma and plasma fraction transfusions

NURSING CONSIDERATIONS

- ABO compatibility is required. Rh-type match not required.
- Use blood administration set and administer as rapidly as tolerated.
- Large-volume transfusions of FFP may require correction for hypocalcemia. Citric acid in FFP binds calcium.

- ABO compatability isn't necessary.
- Use the administration set supplied by the manufacturer; rate and volume depend on the patient's condition and response.
- Reactions to albumin (fever, chills, nausea) are rare.
- Albumin shouldn't be mixed with protein hydrolysates and alcohol solutions.
- Albumin is commonly given as a volume expander until crossmatching for whole blood is complete.
- Albumin is contraindicated as an expander in severe anemia; administer cautiously in patients with cardiac and pulmonary disease because of the risk of heart failure from circulatory overload.

- ABO compatibility isn't necessary but is preferable.
- Use the manufacturer-supplied administration set; administer with a filter. Standard dose recommended for treatment of acute bleeding episodes in hemophilia is 15 to 20 units/kg.
- Half-life of factor VIII (8 to 10 hours) necessitates repeat transfusions at these intervals to maintain normal levels.
- Administer I.V. as rapidly as tolerated, but don't exceed 6 ml/minute; monitor pulse rate while infusing.

- No ABO or Rh matching is necessary.
- Use a straight-line set; dosage is based on desired level and the patient's body weight.
- Risk of hepatitis is high.
- Coagulation assays are performed before administration and at suitable intervals during treatment.
- Administration is contraindicated when the patient has liver disease resulting in fibrinolysis.
- Administration is contraindicated when the patient has intravascular coagulation and isn't undergoing heparin therapy.

Complex transfusions

Specialized methods for administering blood include autotransfusion and hemiparesis. Both methods must be performed by skilled personnel. Only nurses who are familiar with the procedures should monitor and evaluate a patient's condition throughout the transfusion.

Autotransfusion is the process of collecting, filtering, and reinfusing the patient's own blood. Many patients prefer autotransfusion because it eliminates the risk of infectious disease. They can begin giving blood 4 to 6 weeks before surgery; the units are collected, tested, labeled, and stored until needed. Blood can also be collected during surgery. It's treated with an anticoagulant and collected in a sterile container that's fitted with a filter. The blood is reinfused as whole blood or processed before infusion. Salvaged blood can't be stored because the filtering and processing can't remove bacteria completely. Hemiparesis is the process of collecting and removing specific blood components and then returning the remaining components to the donor.

TRANSFUSIONS FOR SPECIAL POPULATIONS

Pediatric and elderly patients require special care during transfusion therapy. For instance, transfusing blood into a neonate requires specialized skills because the neonate's physiologic requirements differ vastly from those of an older infant, child, adolescent, or adult.

Children

Transfusions in children differ from transfusions in adults significantly:
- Blood units for children are prepared in half-unit packs, and a 24G or 22G thin-walled catheter is used to administer the blood.
- Usually, a child receives 5% to 10% of the total transfusion in the first 15 minutes of therapy. To maintain the correct infusion rate, an electronic infusion device should be used.
- A child's normal circulating blood volume determines the amount of blood transfused. The average blood volume for children and infants older than age 1 month is 75 ml/kg. The proportion of blood volume to body weight decreases with age.
- Whenever an infant or child is receiving a blood transfusion, the procedure, its purpose, and the possible complications should be explained to the parents or legal guardian. If appropriate, the

child should also be included in the explanation. The parents should be asked about the child's transfusion history, and their consent should be obtained for transfusion.
- The child should be closely monitored, particularly during the first 15 minutes to detect early signs of a reaction. A blood warmer should be used, if indicated, to prevent hypothermia and cardiac arrhythmias, especially when administering blood through a central line.
- In massive hemorrhage and shock, the indications for blood component transfusion in children remain similar to those for adults, although accurate assessment is difficult. Blood drawn from a central vein provides more accurate hemoglobin (Hb) and hematocrit measurements, or blood pressure readings are used to assess blood volume.

Elderly patients

An elderly patient with preexisting heart disease may be unable to tolerate rapid transfusion of an entire unit of blood without exhibiting shortness of breath or other signs of heart failure. The patient may be better able to tolerate half-unit blood transfusions.

Age-related slowing of the immune system puts an older adult at risk for delayed transfusion reactions. Because greater quantities of blood products transfuse before signs or symptoms appear, the patient may experience a more severe reaction. Also, an elderly patient tends to be less resistant to infection.

COMPLICATIONS

Always take steps to prevent transfusion complications, and know how they are managed when they arise. (See *Correcting transfusion problems,* page 220.)

Transfusion reactions

Usually attributed to major antigen-antibody reactions, transfusion reactions may occur up to 4 days after the transfusion begins. Transfusion reactions occur more commonly with the administration of platelets, white blood cells (WBCs), and cryoprecipitate than with whole blood, red blood cells (RBCs), or plasma.

Whenever signs or symptoms of an acute transfusion reaction are detected, the transfusion should be stopped immediately. These steps are followed:
- The I.V. tubing should be changed to prevent infusing more blood. The blood tubing and bag should be saved for analysis.
- Normal saline solution should be given to keep the vein patent (open).

> **BEST PRACTICE**
>
> ## Correcting transfusion problems
>
> A patient who receives excellent care can still encounter problems during a transfusion. Your state nurse practice and facility policy may not permit you to perform or assist with correcting these problems, however, you should know about them. Here's what should be done when common transfusion problems occur.
>
> ### IT STOPPED!
> If the transfusion stops, these steps should be followed:
> - The I.V. container should be at least 3′ (1 m) above the level of the I.V. site.
> - The infusion clamp is opened.
> - The blood completely covers the filter. If it doesn't, the drip chamber is squeezed until it does.
> - The bag is gently rocked back and forth, so that blood cells that may have settled on the bottom are agitated.
> - If a Y-type blood administration set is used, the flow clamp to the patient is closed and the blood bag lowered. Next, the normal saline solution line clamp is opened and the solution is allowed to flow into the blood bag. The blood bag should be rehung, the flow clamp to the patient opened, and the flow rate reset.
>
> ### HEMATOMA
> If a hematoma develops at the I.V. site, these steps should be followed:
> - The infusion is immediately stopped.
> - The needle or catheter should be removed and the tubing should be capped with a new needleless connection.
> - The physician should be notified and ice placed on the site for 24 hours; after that, warm compresses are applied.
> - Reabsorption of the hematoma should be encouraged by having the patient gently exercise the affected limb.
> - Observations and actions are documented.
>
> ### AN EMPTY BAG
> If the blood bag empties before the next one arrives when a Y-type set is used, these steps are followed:
> - The blood-line clamp is closed.
> - The normal saline solution-line clamp is opened.
> - The normal saline solution should run slowly until the new blood arrives.
> - The flow rate should be decreased or the line clamped before attaching the new unit of blood.

- The patient's vital signs should be taken and recorded.
- The physician should be notified.
- A urine specimen and blood sample should be obtained and sent to the laboratory.
- Further treatment should be prepared for.

- A transfusion reaction report and an incident report should be completed according to your facility's policies and procedures.
- The physician or blood bank may eliminate some of these steps if a patient has a history of frequent mild reactions.

Transfusion of blood products that have been processed and preserved increases the patient's risk of complications, especially if the patient receives frequent transfusions of large amounts. Hemolytic, febrile, and allergic reactions can follow any transfusion. (See *Managing transfusion reactions,* pages 222 to 225.)

HEMOLYTIC REACTIONS
An acute hemolytic reaction is life-threatening. It occurs as a result of incompatible blood or improper blood storage. A hemolytic reaction almost always results from a clerical error, such as mislabeling or failing to properly identify the patient, and may progress to shock and renal failure.

FEBRILE REACTIONS
Nonhemolytic febrile reactions are characterized by a temperature increase of 1.8° F (1° C). Such reactions are related to a transfusion and aren't caused by disease. Febrile reactions usually result from the patient's anti-human leukocyte antigen antibodies reacting against antigens on the donor's WBCs or platelets. Febrile reactions occur in 1% of transfusions, immediately or within 2 hours after transfusion.

Signs and symptoms of febrile reactions include:
- chest pain
- chills
- dyspnea
- fever
- headache
- hypotension
- malaise
- nausea and vomiting
- nonproductive cough.

ALLERGIC REACTIONS
An allergic reaction is the second most common transfusion reaction. It occurs because of an allergen in the transfused blood. Signs of an allergic reaction may include:
- chills
- face swelling

(Text continues on page 232.)

BEST PRACTICE

Managing transfusion reactions

If the patient experiences a transfusion reaction, the infusion should be stopped and this table consulted for further steps and tips for preventing reactions when restarting.

REACTION	NURSING INTERVENTIONS
REACTIONS FROM ANY TRANSFUSION	
Hemolytic	• Blood pressure should be monitored. • Shock should be treated as indicated by the patient's condition, using I.V. fluids, oxygen, epinephrine, a diuretic, and a vasopressor. • Post-transfusion reaction blood and urine samples should be obtained for evaluation. • The patient should be observed for signs of hemorrhage resulting from disseminated intravascular coagulation.
Febrile	• Symptoms can be relieved with an antipyretic or antihistamine.
Allergic	• An antihistamine should be given. • The patient should be monitored for an anaphylactic reaction and epinephrine and steroids given, if indicated.
Plasma protein incompatibility	• Shock should be treated by administering oxygen, fluids, epinephrine and, possibly, a steroid.
Bacterial contamination	• A broad-spectrum antibiotic and a steroid should be given.
Circulation overload	• The transfusion should be stopped. • The I.V. should be maintained with normal saline solution. • Oxygen should be given. • The patient's head should be elevated. • A diuretic should be given, if ordered.

Prevention

- Before the transfusion is restarted, the donor and recipient blood types should be rechecked to ensure blood compatibility; the patient should be identified with another nurse or a physician in the room.
- Blood should be transfused slowly for the first 15 to 20 minutes; the patient should be closely observe for the first 30 minutes of the transfusion.

- An antipyretic, an antihistamine and, possibly, a steroid should be used to premedicate.
- Leukocyte-poor or washed red blood cells (RBCs) should be used. A leukocyte removal filter specific to the component should be used.

- If the patient has a history of allergic reactions, an antihistamine should be used to premedicate.
- The patient should be observed closely for the first 30 minutes of the transfusion.

- Only immunoglobulin A-deficient blood or well-washed RBCs should be transfused.

- Blood should be inspected before the transfusion for gas, clots, and a dark purple color.
- Air-free, touch-free methods should be used to draw and deliver blood.
- Strict storage control should be maintained.
- The blood tubing and filter should be changed every 4 hours.
- Each unit of blood should be infused over 2 to 4 hours; if the infusion exceeds 4 hours, stop it.
- Sterile technique should be maintained.

- Blood should be transfused slowly.
- No more than 2 units in 4 hours should be given, fewer for elderly patients, infants, or patients with cardiac conditions.

(continued)

Managing transfusion reactions (continued)

REACTION	NURSING INTERVENTIONS
REACTIONS FROM MULTIPLE TRANSFUSIONS	
Hemosiderosis	• A phlebotomy should be done to remove excess iron.
Bleeding tendencies	• Platelets should be given. • Platelet count should be monitored.
Elevated blood ammonia level	• The ammonia level should be monitored. • Protein in the diet should be decreased. • Lactulose (Cephulac) should be given, if indicated.
Increased oxygen affinity for hemoglobin	• The arterial blood gas level should be monitored and respiratory support given as needed.
Hypothermia	• The transfusion should be stopped. • The patient should be warmed with blankets. • An electrocardiogram (ECG) should be obtained.
Hypocalcemia	• Potassium and calcium levels should be monitored. • If multiple units are being given, blood less than 2 days old should be used. • The transfusion should be slowed or stopped, depending on the reaction. Hypothermic patients or patients with elevated potassium levels may have a worse reaction. • I.V. calcium gluconate should be given slowly.
Potassium intoxication	• An ECG should be taken. • Sodium polystyrene sulfonate (Kayexalate) should be given orally or by enema.

- fever
- hives
- itching
- throat swelling
- wheezing.

An allergic reaction may progress to an anaphylactic reaction. This reaction can occur immediately or within 1 hour after infusion.

Prevention

- Blood should be given only when absolutely necessary.

- Only fresh blood less than 7 days old should be used, if possible.

- Only RBCs, fresh frozen plasma, or fresh blood should be used, especially if the patient has liver disease.

- Only RBCs or fresh blood should be used, if possible.

- The blood should be warmed to 95° to 98° F (35° to 36.7° C), especially for a massive transfusion.

- Blood should be given slowly.

- Fresh blood should be used when giving a massive transfusion.

Severe anaphylactic reactions produce bronchospasm, dyspnea, pulmonary edema, and hypotension. Treatment includes immediate administration of epinephrine, corticosteroids, and antihistamines. Provide necessary respiratory support or cardiopulmonary resuscitation, if needed.

Other common complications may come up. (See *Common transfusion complications,* page 226.) Knowing about them and their

Common transfusion complications

PLASMA PROTEIN INCOMPATIBILITY
Plasma protein incompatibility usually results from blood that contains immunoglobulin (Ig) A proteins being infused into an IgA-deficient recipient who has developed anti-IgA antibodies. The reaction can be life-threatening and usually resembles anaphylaxis. Signs and symptoms include:
- flushing and urticaria
- abdominal pain
- chills
- fever
- dyspnea and wheezing
- hypotension
- shock
- cardiac arrest.

BACTERIAL CONTAMINATION
Blood and blood products may be contaminated during the collection process. As storage times and temperature increase, the growth of microorganisms also increases. The resulting transfusion reaction is most commonly related to the endotoxins produced by gram-negative bacteria. Signs and symptoms of bacterial contamination include:
- chills
- fever
- vomiting
- abdominal cramping
- diarrhea
- shock
- kidney failure.

signs and symptoms will give you confidence to deal with them when they arise.

Multiple-transfusion reactions

Certain complications typically result from multiple or massive transfusions. These include:
- bleeding tendencies
- elevated blood ammonia levels
- hemosiderosis (accumulation of an iron-containing protein)
- hypocalcemia
- hypothermia
- increased oxygen affinity for Hb
- potassium intoxication.

HEMOSIDEROSIS
Accumulation of an iron-containing pigment (hemosiderin) may be associated with RBC destruction in a patient who receives many transfusions. In hemosiderosis, the patient's iron level is greater than 200 mg/dl.

BLEEDING TENDENCIES
A low platelet count — which can develop in stored blood — can cause bleeding tendencies. Signs and symptoms may include abnormal bleeding, oozing from a cut or break in the skin surface, and abnormal clotting values.

ELEVATED AMMONIA LEVEL
Ammonia levels can increase in a patient receiving a transfusion of stored blood. Signs and symptoms of high ammonia levels include forgetfulness and confusion. The patient may also have a sweet mouth odor. High ammonia levels can cause behaviors that range from stuporlike to combative.

INCREASED OXYGEN AFFINITY FOR HEMOGLOBIN
A blood transfusion can cause a decreased level of 2,3-diphosphoglycerate (2,3-DPG). Found on RBCs but scarce in stored blood, 2,3-DPG affects the oxyhemoglobin dissociation curve. This curve represents Hb saturation and desaturation in graph form. Levels of 2,3-DPG, as well as other factors, cause the curve to shift either to the right (causing a decrease in oxygen affinity) or to the left (causing an increase in oxygen affinity).

When 2,3-DPG levels are low, they produce a shift to the left. This causes an increase in oxygen affinity for Hb, so the oxygen stays in the patient's bloodstream and isn't released into other tissues. Signs of this reaction include a depressed respiratory rate, especially in the patient with chronic lung disease.

HYPOTHERMIA
A rapid infusion of large amounts of cold blood can cause hypothermia. The patient may experience shaking chills, hypotension, and cardiac arrhythmias, which may become life-threatening. Cardiac arrest can occur if the patient's core temperature falls below 86° F (30° C).

HYPOCALCEMIA
If blood is infused too rapidly, citrate toxicity can occur. (Citrate is used to preserve blood.) Because citrate binds with calcium, calcium deficiency may result. Toxicity may also follow normal citrate metabolism that's hindered by a liver disorder. Signs and symptoms of calcium deficiency include:
- tingling in the fingers
- muscle cramps
- nausea

- vomiting
- hypotension
- cardiac arrhythmias
- seizures.

POTASSIUM INTOXICATION
Some cells in stored RBCs may leak potassium into the plasma. Intoxication usually doesn't occur with a transfusion of 1 or 2 units of blood, but larger volumes may cause potassium toxicity. Signs and symptoms of potassium toxicity may include:
- irritability
- intestinal colic
- diarrhea
- muscle weakness
- oliguria
- renal failure
- electrocardiogram changes with tall, peaked T waves
- bradycardia that may proceed to cardiac arrest.

TRANSMISSION OF DISEASE
Unlike a transfusion reaction, an infectious disease transmitted during a transfusion may go undetected until days, weeks, or months later, when signs and symptoms appear. Remember, all blood products are potential carriers of infectious disease, including:
- hepatitis
- human immunodeficiency virus (HIV)
- cytomegalovirus (CMV).

Steps to prevent disease transmission include laboratory testing of blood products and careful screening of potential donors. Neither of these precautions is foolproof. Hepatitis C (non-A, non-B) accounts for most posttransfusion hepatitis cases. The test that detects hepatitis C can produce false-negative results and may allow some contamination to go undetected. HIV screening determines the presence of antibodies and antigens to HIV. The Food and Drug Administration requires that the antigen test be used in conjunction with the antibody test to reduce the risk of exposure from blood transfusions. False-negative results can occur, particularly during the incubation period of about 6 to 12 weeks after exposure. The Centers for Disease Control and Prevention estimates that undetected infection occurs in 1 out of every 450,000 to 660,000 donations per year. Many facilities screen blood for CMV. Blood with CMV is especially dangerous for an immunosuppressed patient.

6

CHEMOTHERAPY INFUSIONS

Understanding I.V. chemotherapy

Chemotherapy, surgery, and radiation are the mainstays of cancer treatment. Chemotherapy is most commonly administered I.V., using peripheral or central veins—although it's also administered by the oral, subcutaneous, intrathecal, I.M., intra-arterial, and intracavitary routes.

Chemotherapy drugs may be administered in the physician's office, in an outpatient clinic, in the patient's home, or in a long-term care facility or hospital. Wherever treatments take place, the same basic principles of I.V. therapy apply. Because of rapid changes in health care delivery, leading to a rise in chemotherapy administration outside the hospital setting, there's an increased emphasis on patient teaching.

Suppressing rapidly dividing cancer cells with chemotherapy requires effective delivery of an exact dose of these toxic drugs. This can be achieved by I.V. chemotherapy. Additional benefits include complete absorption and systemic distribution.

While chemotherapy is intended to control or eliminate cancer cells, it can also damage healthy cells. Healthy cells are attacked because the chemotherapy can't differentiate between healthy and cancerous cells. Chemotherapy attacks all rapidly growing cells. Two examples of rapidly growing cells are hair and nail follicles—this is why patients lose their hair and why their nails become brittle.

Frequent I.V. chemotherapy use can lead veins to become sclerotic. Chemotherapy patients are also at risk for phlebitis or tissue necrosis.

HOW CHEMOTHERAPY WORKS

Healthy and cancerous cells pass through similar life cycles and are similarly vulnerable to chemotherapeutic drugs. Some of these drugs are cycle-specific — designed to disrupt a specific biochemical process, making them effective only during specific phases of the cell cycle. Other drugs are cycle-nonspecific, meaning that their prolonged action is independent of the cell cycle, allowing them to act on reproducing and resting cells.

Because tumor cells are active in various phases of the cell cycle, chemotherapy typically employs more than one drug. This way, each drug can target a different site or take action during a different phase of the cell cycle.

During a single administration of a cycle-nonspecific chemotherapeutic drug, a fixed percentage of normal and malignant cells die, while a percentage of normal and malignant cells survive.

When cycle-specific chemotherapy is given, cells in the resting phase survive. (See *The cell cycle and chemotherapeutic drugs*.)

The challenge is to provide a drug dose large enough to kill the greatest number of cancer cells but small enough to avoid irreversibly damaging normal tissue or causing toxicity. Given together, the drugs increase each other's actions, and the tumor responds as it would to a larger dose of a single drug.

In addition, because different drugs work at different stages of the cell cycle or employ different mechanisms to kill cancer cells, using several drugs decreases the likelihood that the tumor will develop resistance to the chemotherapy.

Which drugs should be part of the regimen?

Drug selection depends on the patient's age, overall condition, tumor type, and allergies or sensitivities as well as the stage of the cancer. Physicians strive to select the most effective drugs for the first round of chemotherapy because this is when cancer cells respond best. Second- or third-line chemotherapy drugs may have to be used, depending on any hypersensitivity reaction the patient may have.

Eradicating a tumor calls for repeated drug doses. This is considered a single course of chemotherapy and is repeated on a cyclic basis. The cycle can be repeated daily, weekly, every other week, or every 3 to 4 weeks. Treatment cycles are carefully planned so normal cells can regenerate. The timing of repeat treatment cycles depends on the cycle of the targeted cells and the return of normal blood counts.

Most patients require at least three treatment cycles before they show a beneficial response. However, every patient differs. Some patients show faster tumor response time than others and some don't respond at all.

The cell cycle and chemotherapeutic drugs

All cells cycle through five phases. Chemotherapeutic drugs that are active on cells during one or more of these phases are called cycle-specific. The illustration tells what happens at each phase of the cell cycle and gives examples of cycle-specific drugs that are active during each phase.

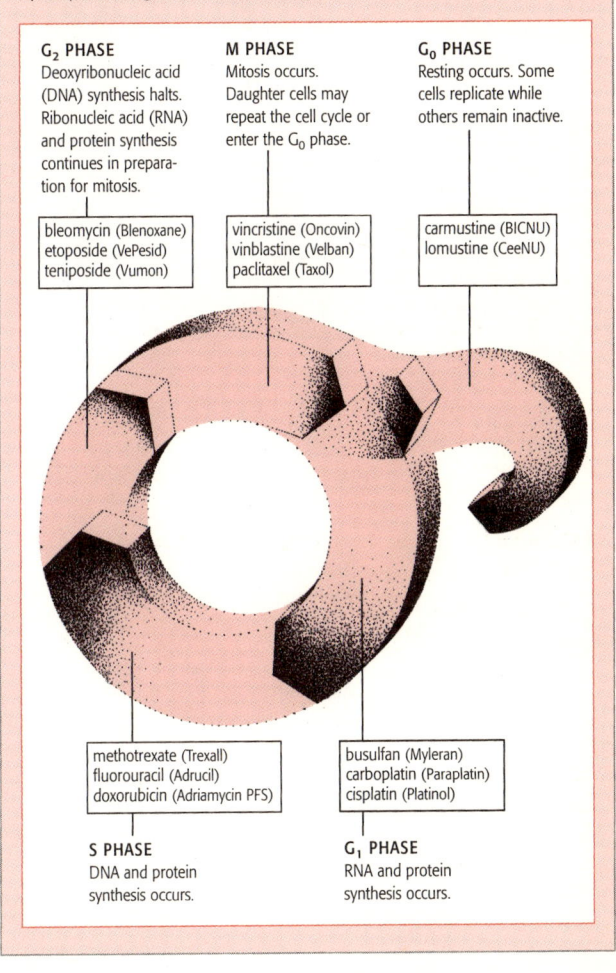

G_2 PHASE
Deoxyribonucleic acid (DNA) synthesis halts. Ribonucleic acid (RNA) and protein synthesis continues in preparation for mitosis.

- bleomycin (Blenoxane)
- etoposide (VePesid)
- teniposide (Vumon)

M PHASE
Mitosis occurs. Daughter cells may repeat the cell cycle or enter the G_0 phase.

- vincristine (Oncovin)
- vinblastine (Velban)
- paclitaxel (Taxol)

G_0 PHASE
Resting occurs. Some cells replicate while others remain inactive.

- carmustine (BICNU)
- lomustine (CeeNU)

S PHASE
DNA and protein synthesis occurs.

- methotrexate (Trexall)
- fluorouracil (Adrucil)
- doxorubicin (Adriamycin PFS)

G_1 PHASE
RNA and protein synthesis occurs.

- busulfan (Myleran)
- carboplatin (Paraplatin)
- cisplatin (Platinol)

Chemotherapeutic drugs

Chemotherapeutic drugs are categorized according to their pharmacologic action as well as the way in which they interfere with cell production. Cycle-specific drugs are divided into:
- antimetabolites

Selected chemotherapeutic drugs

Compare the characteristics and toxic effects of these chemotherapeutic drugs.

DRUG TYPE	CHARACTERISTICS	TOXIC EFFECTS
CYCLE-SPECIFIC		
ANTIMETABOLITES cytarabine (Cytosar-U), floxuridine (FUDR), fluorouracil (Adrucil), hydroxyurea (Hydrea), methotrexate (Trexall), thioguanine (Tabloid)	• Interfere with nucleic acid synthesis • Attack during S phase of cell cycle	• Effects on bone marrow (myelosuppression), central nervous system (CNS), and GI system
PLANT ALKALOIDS vinblastine (Velban), vincristine (Oncovin)	• Prevent mitotic spindle formation • Cycle-specific to M phase	• Effects on CNS and GI system • Myelosuppression • Tissue damage
ENZYMES asparaginase (Elspar)	• Useful only in leukemias	• Hypersensitivity reactions
CYCLE-NONSPECIFIC		
ALKYLATING DRUGS carboplatin (Paraplatin), cisplatin (Platinol), cyclophosphamide (Cytoxan), ifosfamide (Ifex), thiotepa (Thioplex)	• Disrupt deoxyribonucleic acid (DNA) replication	• Infertility • Secondary carcinoma • Effects on renal system
ANTIBIOTIC ANTINEOPLASTICS bleomycin (Blenoxane), doxorubicin (Adriamycin PFS), idarubicin (Idamycin), mitoxantrone (Novantrone), mitomycin (Mutamycin)	• Bind with DNA to inhibit synthesis of DNA and ribonucleic acid	• Effects on GI, renal, and hepatic systems • Effects on bone marrow

- plant alkaloids.

Cycle-nonspecific drugs are divided into:
- alkylating agents
- nitrosoureas
- antineoplastics
- antibiotic antineoplastics
- miscellaneous.

Other drugs used to inhibit tumor-cell growth include steroids, hormones, and antihormones. These drugs work in the intracellular environment. Steroids, which normally act as anti-inflammatory agents, make malignant cells vulnerable to damage from cell-specific drugs. Hormones alter the environment of cells by affecting the permeability of their membranes. Antihormones affect hormone-dependent tumors by inhibiting the production of those hormones or neutralizing their effects. (See *Selected chemotherapeutic drugs*.)

Physicians order chemotherapeutic drugs to control cancer, to cure cancer, to prevent metastasis, or for palliative care. Drugs may

Selected chemotherapeutic drugs *(continued)*

CATEGORY	CHARACTERISTICS	TOXIC EFFECTS
HORMONES AND HORMONE INHIBITORS		
androgens (testolactone [Teslac]), anti-androgens (flutamide [Eulexin]), anti-estrogens (tamoxifen [Nolvadex]), estrogens (estramustine [Emcyt]), gonadotropins (leuprolide [Lupron]), progestins (megestrol [Megace])	• Interfere with binding of normal hormones to receptor proteins, manipulate hormone levels, and alter hormone environment • Mechanism of action not always clear • Usually palliative, not curative	• No known toxic effect
FOLIC ACID ANALOGS		
leucovorin (Wellcovorin)	• Antidote for methotrexate toxicity	• Hypersensitivity reaction possible
CYTOPROTECTIVE DRUGS		
dexrazoxane (Zinecard), mesna (MESNEX)	• Protect normal tissue by binding with metabolites of other cytotoxic drugs	• None

Sample chemotherapy protocols

Chemotherapeutic drugs are commonly given in combinations called protocols. Here are the protocols typically given for some common cancers.

CANCERS	PROTOCOLS	DRUGS
Bladder cancer	CISCA	• cisplatin (Platinol) • cyclophosphamide (Cytoxan) • Adriamycin (doxorubicin)
Breast cancer	AC	• Adriamycin (doxorubicin) • cyclophosphamide (Cytoxan)
Cervical cancer	MOBP	• mitomycin (Mutamycin) • Oncovin (vincristine) • bleomycin (Blenoxane) • Platinol (cisplatin)
Prostate cancer	FL	• flutamide (Eulexin) • leuprolide (Lupron)
Gastric cancer	EAP	• etoposide (VePesid) • Adriamycin (doxorubicin) • Platinol (cisplatin)
Head and neck cancer	CF	• cisplatin (Platinol) • fluorouracil (Adrucil)
Acute lymphocytic leukemia, induction	DVP	• daunorubicin (Cerubidine) • vincristine (Oncovin) • prednisone (Deltasone)
Melanoma	CPB	• cisplatin (Platinol) • procarbazine (Matulane) • BICNU (carmustine)
Acute myelocytic leukemia, consolidation	MC	• mitoxantrone (Novantrone) • cytarabine (Cytosar-U)
Lymphoma (non-Hodgkin's)	CVP (COP)	• cyclophosphamide (Cytoxan) • vincristine (Oncovin) • prednisone (Deltasone)

Sample chemotherapy protocols *(continued)*

CANCERS	PROTOCOLS	DRUGS
Lung cancer, small-cell	CAE (ACE)	• cyclophosphamide (Cytoxan) • Adriamycin (doxorubicin) • etoposide (VePesid)
Lung cancer, non-small-cell	CAP	• cyclophosphamide (Cytoxan) • Adriamycin (doxorubicin) • Platinol (cisplatin)
Lymphoma (Hodgkin's disease)	ABVD	• Adriamycin (doxorubicin) • bleomycin (Blenoxane) • vinblastine (Velban) • dacarbazine (DTIC-Dome)
Lymphoma, malignant	BEACOPP	• bleomycin (Blenoxane) • etoposide (VePesid) • Adriamycin (doxorubicin) • cyclophosphamide (Cytoxan) • Oncovin (vincristine) • procarbazine (Matulane) • prednisone (Deltasone) • filgrastim (Neupogen)
Multiple myeloma	MP	• melphalan (Alkeran) • prednisone (Deltasone)
Testicular cancer	BEP	• bleomycin (Blenoxane) • etoposide (VePesid) • Platinol (cisplatin)

be given alone or in combinations, called *protocols*. (See *Sample chemotherapy protocols*.)

The search for new cancer treatments is ongoing. Each year, the National Cancer Institute screens about 15,000 potential new compounds for chemotherapeutic action. Specific areas of research include biological therapy and immunotherapy.

Immunotherapy

In cancer immunotherapy, drugs known as biological response modifiers are used to enhance the body's ability to destroy cancer cells.

Cancer immunotherapy seeks to evoke effective immune response to human tumors by altering the way cells grow, mature, and respond to cancer cells. This approach is unique because it manipulates the body's natural resources instead of introducing toxic substances that aren't selective and can't differentiate between normal or abnormal processes or cells. Immunotherapy may include the administration of monoclonal antibodies and immunomodulatory cytokines.

MONOCLONAL ANTIBODIES

Monoclonal antibodies, which specifically target tumor cells, are a relatively new form of immunotherapy.

Antibodies are immunoglobulins produced by mature B cells or plasma cells in response to antigens—proteins found on the surface of normal and abnormal cells. Antibodies recognize specific antigens and bind exclusively to them; this process is referred to as a lock-and-key mechanism. When these antibodies attach to antigens, they can cause tumor-cell inactivation or destruction. A monoclonal antibody recognizes only a single unique antigen.

Three monoclonal antibodies have been approved by the Food and Drug Administration for cancer therapy:
- rituximab (Rituxan)
- trastuzumab (Herceptin)
- bevacizumab (Avastin)

Rituxan is specifically indicated for relapsed or refractory low-grade Hodgkin's disease and non-Hodgkin's lymphoma.

Trastuzumab is beneficial against metastatic breast cancer. This monoclonal antibody may be used as a first-line treatment in combination with chemotherapy or as a second-line single agent.

Bevacizumab is used in patients with metastatic colon cancer. It's the first monoclonal antibody that prevents the formation of new blood vessels so that tumor cells don't receive blood, oxygen, and other nutrients needed for growth.

IMMUNOMODULATORY CYTOKINES

Immunomodulatory cytokines are intracellular messenger proteins (proteins that deliver messages within cells). These proteins include:
- interferon alpha

- interleukins
- tumor necrosis factor (TNF)
- colony-stimulating factors (CSFs).

Interferon alpha
Interferon alpha has antiviral and antitumorigenic effects. It slows cell replication and stimulates an immune response. Interferon alpha is approved for treating chronic myeloid leukemia, hairy cell leukemia, and acquired immunodeficiency syndrome-related Kaposi's sarcoma. It's also used with low-grade malignant lymphoma, multiple myeloma, and renal cell carcinoma.

Interleukins
Interleukins are cytokines that primarily function to deliver messages to leukocytes. Interleukin-2 (IL-2) is an approved anticancer agent. IL-2 stimulates the proliferation and cytolytic activity of T cells and natural killer cells. High doses of IL-2 have been effective in a few patients with metastatic renal cell carcinoma and melanoma. The other interleukins remain under investigation for cancer therapy.

Tumor necrosis factor
TNF plays a role in the inflammatory response to tumors and cancer cells. In animal studies, TNF has sometimes produced impressive antitumor responses. This drug is considered investigational.

Colony-stimulating factors
CSFs are substances that are naturally produced by the body. They stimulate the growth of different types of cells found in blood and the immune system. CSFs have been helpful in the clinical care of patients receiving myelosuppressive therapy. Examples of CSFs include:
- Erythropoietin (Epogen, Procrit) induces erythroid maturation (maturation of red blood cells [RBCs]) and increases the release of reticulocytes from the bone marrow—this stimulates RBC production, which may reduce the number of blood transfusions needed by the patient.
- Granulocyte CSF (filgrastim [Neupogen]) stimulates proliferation, differentiation, and functioning of neutrophils, causing a rapid rise in the white blood cell count. Granulocyte CSF is given to reduce the incidence of infection in patients receiving chemotherapy drugs.

- Granulocyte-macrophage CSF (sargramostim [Leukine]) is indicated for older patients receiving chemotherapy for acute myelogenous leukemia, for patients undergoing bone marrow transplants, and for peripheral blood progenitor collection.

Preparing and giving chemotherapy

Many health care facilities use existing guidelines as a basis for their policies and procedures regarding chemotherapeutic drugs. Among the major sources for these guidelines are the following agencies and associations:
- The American Society of Health-System Pharmacists has published guidelines for the preparation of chemotherapeutic drugs since 1990.
- The Occupational Safety and Health Administration (OSHA) published its revised standards for controlling exposure to chemotherapeutic agents in 1995, and needle-stick protection in 2001.
- The Oncology Nursing Society published guidelines for nursing education, practice, and administration of chemotherapeutic agents in 1999.
- The Infusion Nurses Society published revised standards of practice for safe delivery of chemotherapeutic agents in 2000.

At the local level, most health care facilities require nurses and pharmacists involved in the preparation and delivery of chemotherapeutic drugs to complete a certification program that covers the safe delivery of chemotherapeutic drugs and the care of the patient with cancer.

PREPARING CHEMOTHERAPY

Preparing chemotherapeutic drugs requires adherence to guidelines about:
- drug preparation areas and equipment
- protective clothing
- specific safety measures.

Workspace and equipment

Drug preparation may be performed by a trained nurse, a pharmacist or, in states that allow it, a supervised pharmacy technician.

Chemotherapeutic drugs should be prepared in a well-ventilated workspace. All drug admixing or compounding should be performed within a Class II Biological Safety Cabinet or a vertical

Equipment for chemotherapy drug preparation

These items should be available in the work area when chemotherapy drugs are being prepared:
- the patient's medication order or record
- prescribed drugs
- appropriate diluent (if necessary)
- medication labels
- long-sleeved gown
- chemotherapy gloves
- face shield or goggles and a face mask
- 20G needles
- hydrophobic filter or dispensing pin
- syringes with luer-lock fittings and needles of various sizes
- I.V. tubing with luer-lock fittings
- 70% alcohol
- sterile gauze pads
- plastic bags with "hazardous drug" labels
- sharps disposal container
- hazardous waste container
- chemotherapy spill kit.

laminar airflow hood with a high efficiency particulate air, or HEPA, filter vented to the outside. The hood pulls the aerosolized chemotherapy drug particles away from the compounder. If a Class II Biological Safety Cabinet isn't available, a special respirator should be worn.

The individual preparing the chemotherapy drugs should have close access to a sink, alcohol sponges, and gauze pads as well as OSHA-required chemotherapy hazardous waste containers, sharps containers, and chemotherapy spill kits. (See *Equipment for chemotherapy drug preparation*.)

Hazardous waste containers should be made of puncture-proof, shatter-proof, leak-proof plastic. Chemotherapy waste is usually identified with yellow biohazard labels. All chemotherapy contaminated I.V. bags, tubing, filters, and syringes must be disposed of in approved hazardous waste containers. Red sharps containers are used to dispose all contaminated sharps such as needles.

Clothing

Essential protective clothing includes:
- a cuffed gown
- gloves
- goggles or a face shield.

Gowns should be disposable, water resistant, and lint-free with long sleeves, knitted cuffs, and a closed front. Gloves designed for use with chemotherapeutic drugs should be disposable and made of thick latex or thick non-latex material. They should also be powder-free because powder can carry contamination from the drugs into the surrounding air. Double gloving is an option when the gloves aren't of the best quality. Gloves should be changed whenever a tear or puncture occurs. Hands should be washed before putting on the gloves and after removing them.

Precautions

Care should be taken to protect staff, patients, and the environment from unnecessary exposure to chemotherapeutic drugs. The person preparing the chemotherapy drugs should not leave the drug preparation area while wearing the protective gear that was worn during drug preparation. Eating, drinking, smoking, or applying cosmetics in the drug-preparation area violates OSHA guidelines.

Protective gear should be put on before the individual begins to compound the chemotherapeutic drugs. Before preparing the drugs, the work area inside the cabinet should be cleaned with 70% alcohol and a disposable towel; the same should be done after the preparer is finished and after a spill. The towel should be discarded into the yellow leak-proof chemotherapy waste container.

If a chemotherapy drug comes in contact with skin, the skin should be washed thoroughly with soap and water to prevent drug absorption. If the drug comes in contact with the eye, it should immediately be flooded with water or isotonic eyewash for at least 5 minutes while holding the eyelid open.

After an accidental exposure, the supervisor should be notified immediately and the individual may be sent to employee health, where the exposure event will be documented in the employee's health record.

Here are some other safety precautions to keep in mind:
- Aseptic technique should be used when all drugs are prepared.
- Blunt-ended needles should be used whenever possible.
- Needles with a hydrophobic filter should be used to remove solutions from vials.
- Vent vials with a hydrophobic filter or use the negative pressure technique to reduce the amount of aerosolized drugs.
- When an ampule is broken, a gauze pad should be wrapped around the neck of the vial to decrease the chances of droplet contamination and glove puncture.
- A face mask and goggles should be worn for protection against splashes and aerosolized drugs.
- Place all contaminated needles in the sharps container, and don't recap needles.

> **BEST PRACTICE**
>
> ## Inside a chemotherapy spill kit
>
> A chemotherapy spill kit should contain:
> - a long-sleeved gown that's water-resistant and nonpermeable, with cuffs and a back closure
> - shoe covers
> - two pairs of powder-free surgical gloves (for double gloving)
> - a respirator mask
> - chemical splash goggles
> - a disposable dustpan and plastic scraper (for collecting broken glass)
> - plastic-backed absorbent towels, or spill-control pillows
> - desiccant powder or granules (for absorbing wet contents)
> - disposable sponges
> - two large cytotoxic waste disposal bags.

- Only syringes and I.V. sets that have a luer-lock fitting should be used.
- All chemotherapeutic drugs should be labeled with a yellow biohazard label.

The prepared chemotherapy drugs should be transported in a sealable plastic bag that's prominently labeled with a yellow chemotherapy biohazard label.

Make sure that your facility's protocols for spills are available in all areas where chemotherapeutic drugs are handled, including patient care areas. Chemotherapy spill kits should be readily available. (See *Inside a chemotherapy spill kit*.)

If a chemotherapy spill occurs, the facility's protocol, which is probably based on OSHA guidelines, should be followed. This protocol will likely follow these steps:

- Protective garments should be put on, if not already wearing them.
- The area should be isolated and the spill contained with absorbent materials from the spill kit.
- A disposable dustpan and scraper should be used to collect any broken glass or desiccant absorbing powder. The dustpan, scraper, and collected spill should be placed in a leakproof, puncture-proof, chemotherapy designated hazardous waste container.
- Aerosolization of the drug should be prevented at all times.
- The spill area should be cleaned with a detergent or bleach solution.

GIVING CHEMOTHERAPY

Because dosage, route, and timing must be exact to avoid possible fatal complications, only chemotherapy-certified nurses should be involved in giving these drugs. It's usually the responsibility of the registered nurse to administer chemotherapy drugs. The role of the licensed practical or vocational nurse is to monitor for adverse reactions, implement nursing actions and care, and patient teaching.

Not only is cancer a frightening and frequently lethal disease, but its treatment brings with it serious risks and fears as well. To give the patient some sense of control in the face of overwhelming odds, explain each procedure you perform and teach him strategies for dealing with fear, pain, and the unwelcome adverse effects of chemotherapy.

Keep in mind that a positive attitude and a strong emotional support system will enable your patient to better endure — if not overcome — the disease and its treatments.

Complications of chemotherapy

The properties that make chemotherapeutic drugs effective in killing cancer cells also make them toxic to normal cells. No organ system is untouched by chemotherapy. All administration protocols strive to time the treatments and adjust the doses in a way that maximizes the effects against cancer cells while allowing time for normal cells to recover between courses of treatment.

Complications resulting from chemotherapy can be categorized according to where or when exposure to the drug began. They're referred to as:
- infusion-site related
- hypersensitivity or anaphylactic reactions
- short-term
- long-term.

INFUSION SITE–RELATED COMPLICATIONS

Infiltration, extravasation, and vein flare reactions are the most common infusion site–related complications. Be sure to document the infusion site–related complication. (See *Documenting infusion site–related complications.*)

Infiltration

Infiltration is the inadvertent leakage of a nonvesicant solution or drug into the surrounding tissue. The main signs are swelling

> **DOCUMENTATION TIPS**
>
> ### Documenting infusion site–related complications
>
> The following information should be recorded:
> - location of the infiltration, vein flare, or extravasation
> - size of the swollen area
> - name of the drug and I.V. solution
> - the patient's complaints
> - nursing interventions
> - time you notified the physician
> - physician's response and orders
> - the patient's response to interventions.

around the I.V. site — this swollen area will be cool to the touch — along with blanching and a change in the I.V. flow rate.

Tightness in the patient's arm — he'll usually complain of numbness and tingling in the swollen area — from large quantities of I.V. solutions entering the tissue indicates a nerve compression injury and can result in compartment syndrome. Notify the physician immediately.

Extravasation

Extravasation is the inadvertent leakage of a vesicant solution (a drug that can cause tissue necrosis and sloughing) into the surrounding tissue.

When the patient is being assessed for extravasation, these considerations should be kept in mind:

- Initial signs of an extravasation may resemble those of infiltration — swelling, pain, and blanching.
- Blood return is an inconclusive test and shouldn't be used to determine if the I.V. catheter is correctly seated in the peripheral vein.
- To assess peripheral I.V. placement, the vein should be flushed with normal saline solution and observed for site swelling.
- Symptoms can progress to blisters; to skin, muscle, tissue, and fat necrosis; and to tissue sloughing. The outer surface of veins, arteries, and nerves can also be damaged. Depending on the drug and the concentration of the drug in the solutions, blistering can be apparent within hours or days of extravasation.
- If anything occurs that causes doubt that the infusion is proceeding as it should, the infusion should be stopped and the venous

Understanding antidotes to vesicant extravasation

This table provides examples of antidotes that may be administered in the event of extravasation by a vesicant. Your state nurse practice act and facility policy may not allow you to give antidotes for extravasation, but it's important that you understand them.

INFILTRATING DRUG	ANTIDOTE	NURSING CONSIDERATIONS
• daunorubicin (Cerubidine) • doxorubicin (Adriamycin PFS)	dimethyl sulfoxide (DMSO)	• Apply a cold pack for at least 1 hour, 4 times per day for 3 to 5 days. • DMSO 50% to 90% solution can be applied to the extravasation site every 6 hours for 14 days. Don't cover the infusion site; allow it to air dry. • Injection of sodium bicarbonate is contraindicated.
• mechlorethamine (nitrogen mustard)	10% sodium thiosulfate	• Sodium thiosulfate is mixed with sterile water for injection and is injected into the existing I.V. line that extravasated. • The catheter is then removed. • The solution may also be given subcutaneously clockwise into the infiltration area. • Apply ice for 6 to 12 hours.

access device removed. Remember, "When in doubt, it should be taken out!"

RED FLAG Always have the extravasation kit readily available and follow the protocol for the specific drug.

If a vesicant has extravasated, it's an emergency. Quickly take the following steps, designed to limit the damage:
- Stop the infusion. Check your facility's policy to determine if the I.V. catheter is to be removed or left in place to infuse corticosteroids or a specific antidote. Treatment for extravasation should be in accordance with the manufacturer's guidelines.
- Notify the physician.
- The appropriate antidote will be given according to facility policy. Usually, an antidote for extravasation is given by either instilling it through the existing I.V. catheter or by using a 1-ml syringe to

subcutaneously inject small amounts in a circle around the extravasated area. After the antidote has been injected, the I.V. catheter is removed. (See *Understanding antidotes to vesicant extravasation*.)
- Continue to visually monitor the site and document its appearance and the patient's response. Subsequent care of the extravasated area may include topical steroids or silver sulfadiazine (Silvadene) cream. If the extravasation injury is severe, the patient may require skin debridement, skin grafts, or possibly amputation.

Vein flare

During infusion of an irritant into the vein, the patient may complain of burning pain or aching along the vein as well as up through the arm. A vein flare (a bright redness) may also appear in the vein along with blotches or hives on the affected arm. If the reaction is severe, injection of an I.V. steroid may be required. In some cases, the infusion of an irritant can result in damage to the lining of the vein wall, causing serious phlebitis or vein thrombosis.

RED FLAG *Irritants require large veins with good hemodilution to decrease the irritating properties of the drug. If the patient complains of pain or burning during the infusion, the dilution of the infused drug should be increased and the infusion rate decreased. The I.V. should be started in a different vein.*

HYPERSENSITIVITY OR ANAPHYLACTIC REACTIONS

Hypersensitivity or anaphylactic reactions can occur at the initial dose of the drug or on subsequent infusions of the same drug. Some chemotherapeutic drugs put the patient at high risk for anaphylaxis:
- asparaginase (Elspar)
- paclitaxel (Taxol)
- rituximab (Rituxan).

These drugs have a moderate to low risk:
- anthracyclines
- bleomycin (Blenoxane)
- carboplatin (Paraplatin)
- cisplatin (Platinol)
- cyclosporine (Neoral)
- etoposide (VePesid)
- melphalan (Alkeran)
- methotrexate (Trexall)
- procarbazine (Matulane)
- teniposide (Vumon).

Signs and symptoms of immediate hypersensitivity

An immediate hypersensitivity reaction to a chemotherapeutic drug will appear within 5 minutes after starting the infusion.

ORGAN SYSTEM	PATIENT COMPLAINT	ASSESSMENT FINDINGS
Respiratory	Dyspnea, inability to speak, tightness in chest	Stridor, bronchospasm, decreased air movement
Skin	Pruritus, urticaria	Cyanosis, urticaria, angioedema, cold, clammy skin
Cardiovascular	Chest pain, increased heart rate	Tachycardia, hypotension, arrhythmias
Central nervous system	Dizziness, agitation, anxiety	Loss of sensation, loss of consciousness

These drugs have a low risk:
- chlorambucil (Leukeran)
- cyclophosphamide (Cytoxan)
- cytarabine (Cytosar-U)
- dacarbazine (DTIC-Dome)
- fluorouracil (Adrucil)
- ifosfamide (Ifex)
- mitoxantrone (Novantrone).

Hypersensitivity reactions can occur at the beginning, middle, or end of the infusion. (See *Signs and symptoms of immediate hypersensitivity*.)

The specific treatment for a hypersensitivity reaction depends on the severity of the reaction. Usually these five steps will be followed:
- The infusion is stopped.
- A rapid infusion of normal saline solution is begun to quickly dilute the drug.
- The patient's vital signs are checked.
- The physician is notified.
- Emergency drugs are given as ordered by the physician.

Antihistamines are typically given first, followed by corticosteroids and bronchodilators. Epinephrine is given first in severe anaphylactic reactions. After you have administered the drug, monitor the patient's vital signs and pulse oximetry every 5 minutes until he's stable, and then every 15 minutes for 1 to 2 hours—or follow facility policy and procedures for acute treatment of allergic reactions.

Throughout the episode, maintain the patient's airway, oxygenation, and tissue perfusion. Life support equipment should be available in case the patient fails to respond. Document the drugs and dosage as well as the patient's response to the treatment.

The patient should discuss future drug infusions with the physician. The physician may reduce the dose of the drug or switch to a drug that targets the tumor type and is less toxic. If the physician continues the drug at a lower dose, premedication with an antihistamine and perhaps a corticosteroid is required. Be sure to check with the physician for preinfusion treatments before subsequent therapy cycles.

SHORT-TERM ADVERSE EFFECTS

The short-term adverse effects of chemotherapy include:
- nausea and vomiting (see *Treating nausea and vomiting related to chemotherapy,* pages 248 and 249.)
- hair loss (alopecia)
- diarrhea
- myelosuppression
- stomatitis.

These effects are produced by damage to tissues with a large proportion of frequently reproducing cells—these tissues include bone marrow, hair follicles, and GI mucosa.

Each patient is different; not all will suffer these adverse effects, and some may not experience any of them.

Alopecia

Alopecia results from the destruction of rapidly dividing cells in the hair shaft or root. It may be minimal or severe, depending on the type of chemotherapy drug and the individual's reaction.

Because so many patients find alopecia disturbing, reassurance about resumed hair growth is important. Inform the patient that his scalp will become sore at times due to the follicles swelling. Educate the patient on hair regrowth. Some patients will have hair growing back during the chemotherapy treatments while others will have no hair growth until 2 to 3 months after treatment is complete. Inform the patient that this new hair may be a different texture or color.

Treating nausea and vomiting related to chemotherapy

Nausea and vomiting can appear in three patterns: anticipatory, acute, and delayed. Each has its own cause. Because daily chemotherapy treatments may last several weeks, expect to see a mix of these three patterns. Managing them is a difficult balancing act but is crucial because of the effects nausea and vomiting have on the patient's nutritional status, emotional well-being, and fluid and electrolyte balance; use this table to help you.

DESCRIPTION	DRUGS	NURSING CONSIDERATIONS
ANTICIPATORY • A learned response from previous nausea and vomiting after a dose of chemotherapy • Most likely to develop in patients with very high anxiety levels who have experienced moderate to severe symptoms after chemotherapy	Lorazepam (Ativan) at least 1 hour before arriving for treatment. Because some patients have overwhelming anxiety, I.V. lorazepam may be needed before chemotherapy is administered.	• Pretreatment is the key. • Posttreatment control can help prevent anticipatory nausea. The less nauseous a patient feels after treatment, the less anxiety he'll experience before the next treatment.
ACUTE • Occur within the first 24 hours of treatment • Cisplatin (Platinol) has a high potential, with more than 90% of patients affected • Bleomycin (Blenoxane) has a low potential, with only 10% to 30% of patients affected • Depends on combination of drugs, doses, infusion rates, and patient characteristics	Aprepitant (Emerol), Ondansetron (Zofran) and granisetron (Kytril). Also lorazepam, dexamethasone (Decadron), metoclopramide (Reglan), and prochlorperazine (Compazine)	• Look for adverse reactions to these drugs.

Treating nausea and vomiting related to chemotherapy (continued)

DESCRIPTION	DRUGS	NURSING CONSIDERATIONS
DELAYED • Loosely defined as starting or continuing beyond 24 hours after chemotherapy has begun • Cause is the least understood of all the types • Has the arsenal of drugs for treating it	In addition to serotonin antagonists and corticosteroids, various antihistamines, benzodiazepines, and metoclopramide	• Look for adverse reactions to these drugs.

Usually a man will wear a ball cap or beret when undergoing chemotherapy. A woman will usually wear a cap, kerchief, or sometimes a wig; tell her to match the wig color up to her natural hair color before total hair loss occurs. The American Cancer Society has helped with the cost of wigs for patients in the past and has even made donated wigs available.

Diarrhea

Diarrhea — brought on because the rapidly dividing cells of the intestinal mucosa are killed — occurs in some patients receiving chemotherapy. Complications of persistent diarrhea include weight loss, fluid and electrolyte imbalance, and malnutrition. To minimize the effects of diarrhea, use dietary adjustments, antidiarrheal medications, and ointments for the rectal area if it's irritated.

Myelosuppression

Myelosuppression is damage to the stem cells in the bone marrow. These cells are the precursors to cellular blood components — red and white blood cells and platelets — so their damage produces anemia, leukopenia, and thrombocytopenia. (See *Managing complications of chemotherapy,* pages 250 and 251.)

BEST PRACTICE

Managing complications of chemotherapy

This table identifies some common adverse effects of chemotherapy and offers ways to minimize them.

ADVERSE EFFECT	SIGNS AND SYMPTOMS	NURSING INTERVENTIONS
Anemia	Dizziness, fatigue, pallor, and shortness of breath after minimal exertion; low hemoglobin (Hb) level and hematocrit (HCT); may develop slowly over several courses of treatment	• Hb level, HCT, and red blood cell count should be monitored, and dropping values should be reported; dehydration from nausea, vomiting, and anorexia causes hemoconcentration, yielding falsely high HCT readings. • A blood transfusion or erythropoietin is given, if needed. • The patient should be told to rest frequently, to increase intake of iron-rich foods, and to take a multivitamin with iron, as prescribed.
Leukopenia	Susceptibility to infections, an absolute neutrophil count less than 1,500 cells/μl	• The *nadir*, the point of lowest blood cell count should be watched for (usually 7 to 14 days after the last treatment). • Colony-stimulating factors should be given. • In the hospitalized patient, neutropenic precautions should be instituted. • The following information should be included in patient and family teaching: good hygiene practices, signs and symptoms of infection, the importance of checking the patient's temperature regularly, how to prepare a low-microbe diet, and how to care for vascular access devices. • The patient should be instructed to avoid crowds, people with colds or respiratory infections, and fresh fruit, fresh flowers, and plants.

Managing complications of chemotherapy
(continued)

ADVERSE EFFECT	SIGNS AND SYMPTOMS	NURSING INTERVENTIONS
Thrombocytopenia	Bleeding gums, increased bruising, petechiae, hypermenorrhea, tarry stools, hematuria, coffee-ground emesis	• Platelet count should be monitored: under 50,000 cells/µl means a moderate risk of excessive bleeding; under 20,000 cells/µl means a major risk and the patient may need a platelet transfusion. • Unnecessary I.M. injections or venipunctures should be avoided; if either is necessary, pressure is applied for at least 5 minutes, and then a pressure dressing is applied to the site. • The patient should be instructed to avoid cuts and bruises, to shave with an electric razor, to avoid blowing his nose, to stay away from irritants that would trigger sneezing, and to not use a rectal thermometer. • The patient should be instructed to report sudden headaches, which could indicate potentially fatal intracranial bleeding.
Alopecia	Hair loss that may include eyebrows, lashes, and body hair	• Shock and distress can be minimized by warning the patient of the possibility of hair loss, discussing why hair loss occurs, and describing how much hair loss to expect. • The need for appropriate head protection against sunburn and heat loss in the winter should be emphasized. • For patients with long hair, cutting the hair shorter before treatment should be recommended because washing and brushing cause more hair loss.

Stomatitis

Stomatitis produces painful mouth ulcers 3 to 7 days after certain chemotherapy drugs are given, with symptoms ranging from mild to severe. Because of the accompanying pain, stomatitis can lead to fluid and electrolyte imbalance and malnutrition if the patient can't swallow or chew adequate food or fluid.

Treat stomatitis with scrupulous oral hygiene and topical anesthetic mixtures. Because pain may be severe, the patient sometimes requires opioid analgesics until ulcers heal. Allow a patient receiving drugs that cause stomatitis to suck on ice chips to help decrease the blood supply to the mouth and decrease ulcer formation.

LONG-TERM ADVERSE EFFECTS

Organ system dysfunction, especially in the hematopoietic and GI systems, is common after chemotherapy. These effects are usually temporary, but some systems suffer permanent damage that manifests itself long after chemotherapy. The renal, pulmonary, cardiac, reproductive, and neurologic systems all show many temporary and permanent dysfunctions from exposure to chemotherapy.

One devastating long-term effect of chemotherapy is secondary malignancy. This can be caused by certain alkylating drugs given for treatment of myeloma, Hodgkin's disease, and malignant lymphomas. A secondary malignancy can occur at any time. The prognosis is usually poor.

7

PARENTERAL NUTRITION

Parenteral nutrition is given when illness or surgery prevents a patient from eating and metabolizing food. Parenteral solutions can provide all the necessary nutrients when a patient can't absorb nutrients through the GI tract. It enables cells to function despite the patient's inability to take in or metabolize food. (See *What parenteral nutrition provides*.)

> ### What parenteral nutrition provides
>
> Essential nutrients found in food provide energy, maintain body tissues, and aid body processes, such as growth, cell activity, enzyme production, and temperature regulation.
>
> When carbohydrates, fats, and proteins are metabolized by the body, they produce energy, which is measured in calories (also called *kilocalories*). A normal healthy adult generally requires 2,000 to 3,000 calories per day. Specific requirements depend on an individual's size, sex, age, and level of physical activity.
>
> A parenteral nutrition solution — also known as *hyperalimentation* or *I.V. hyperalimentation* — may contain one or more of these elements:
> - dextrose
> - proteins
> - lipids
> - electrolytes
> - vitamins
> - trace elements
> - water.

INFUSION METHODS

Depending on the type of therapy ordered, nutritional support solutions are administered through either a central venous (CV) or peripheral infusion device.

Central venous infusion

If a patient needs parenteral nutrition for more than 5 days, he usually requires total parenteral nutrition (TPN). TPN with a final dextrose concentration of 10% or higher must be delivered through a CV line, usually placed in the subclavian vein, with the tip of the catheter in the superior vena cava.

Peripheral infusion

Peripheral parenteral nutrition (PPN)—also called *partial parenteral nutrition*—is the delivery of nutrients through a short catheter inserted into a peripheral vein. Generally, PPN provides fewer nonprotein calories than TPN because lower dextrose concentrations are used. A much larger volume of fluid must be infused for PPN to deliver the same number of calories as TPN. Therefore, most patients who require parenteral nutrition therapy receive TPN, and PPN is reserved for short-term therapy of 1 to 3 weeks.

INDICATIONS

The patient's condition determines whether total parenteral nutrition (TPN) or peripheral parenteral nutrition (PPN) is used. (See *Common conditions that necessitate parenteral nutrition*.)

Indications for total parenteral nutrition

A patient may receive TPN for:
- debilitating illness lasting longer than 2 weeks
- deficient or absent oral intake for longer than 7 days, as in cases of multiple trauma, severe burns, or anorexia nervosa
- loss of at least 10% of pre-illness weight
- serum albumin level below 3.5 g/dl
- poor tolerance of long-term enteral feedings
- chronic vomiting or diarrhea
- inability to sustain adequate weight with oral or enteral feedings
- GI disorders that prevent or severely reduce absorption, such as bowel obstruction, Crohn's disease, ulcerative colitis, short-bowel syndrome, cancer malabsorption syndrome, and bowel fistulas
- inflammatory GI disorders, such as wound infection, fistulas, or abscesses.

Common conditions that necessitate parenteral nutrition

Here's a list of some common conditions and disorders for which the patient may receive parenteral nutrition:
- GI trauma
- pancreatitis
- ileus
- inflammatory bowel disease
- GI tract malignancy
- GI hemorrhage
- paralytic ileus
- GI obstruction
- short-bowel syndrome
- GI fistula
- severe malabsorption.

Indications for peripheral parenteral nutrition

A patient who doesn't need to gain weight, yet needs nutritional support, may receive PPN for as long as 3 weeks. It's used to help a patient meet minimum calorie and protein requirements. PPN may also be used with oral or enteral feedings for a patient who needs to supplement low-calorie intake or who can't absorb enteral therapy.

RED FLAG PPN shouldn't be used for patients with moderate to severe malnutrition or fat metabolism disorders, such as pathologic hyperlipidemia, lipid nephrosis, and acute pancreatitis caused by hyperlipidemia. In patients with severe liver damage, coagulation disorders, anemia, pulmonary disease and in those at increased risk for fat embolism, use parenteral nutrition cautiously.

Nutritional deficiencies

The most common nutritional deficiencies involve protein and calories. Nutritional deficiencies may result from a nonfunctional GI tract, decreased food intake, increased metabolic need, or a combination of these factors.

Food intake may be decreased because of illness, decreased physical ability, or injury. Decreased food intake can occur with GI disorders, such as paralytic ileus, surgery, or sepsis.

An increase in metabolic activity requires an increase in calorie intake. Fever commonly increases metabolic activity. The metabolic rate may also increase in a victim of a burn, trauma, a disease, or stress; a patient may require up to twice the calories of his basal metabolic rate (the minimum energy needed to maintain respiration, circulation, and other basic body functions).

When the body detects protein-calorie deficiency, it turns to its reserve sources of energy. Reserve energy is drawn from three

> ## Consequences of protein-energy malnutrition
>
> - Reduced enzyme and plasma protein production
> - Increased susceptibility to infection
> - Physical and mental growth deficiencies in children
> - Severe diarrhea and malabsorption
> - Numerous secondary nutritional deficiencies
> - Delayed wound healing
> - Mental fatigue

sources. First, the body mobilizes and converts glycogen to glucose through a process called glycogenolysis. Next, if necessary, the body draws energy from the fats stored in adipose tissue. As a last resort, the body taps its store of essential visceral proteins (serum albumin and transferrin) and somatic body proteins (skeletal, smooth muscle, and tissue proteins). These proteins and their amino acids are converted to glucose for energy through a process called gluconeogenesis. The breakdown of these essential body proteins causes a negative nitrogen balance, which means more protein is used by the body than is taken in. Starvation and disease-related stress contribute to this catabolic (destructive) state.

PROTEIN-ENERGY MALNUTRITION

A deficiency of protein and energy (calories) results in protein-energy malnutrition (PEM), also called *protein-calorie malnutrition*. PEM refers to a spectrum of disorders that occur as a result of chronic inadequate protein or calorie intake or high metabolic protein and energy requirements. Protein and energy deficiency can affect every body system. (See *Consequences of protein-energy malnutrition*.)

Disorders that commonly lead to PEM include:
- cancer
- GI disorders
- chronic heart failure
- alcoholism
- conditions causing high metabolic needs such as burns.

PEM takes three basic forms:
- iatrogenic PEM
- kwashiorkor
- marasmus.

Iatrogenic protein-energy malnutrition

During hospitalization, a patient's nutritional status commonly deteriorates because of inadequate protein or calorie intake, leading to iatrogenic PEM. Iatrogenic PEM affects more than 15% of patients in acute care centers. It's most common in patients hospitalized for longer than 2 weeks.

Kwashiorkor

Kwashiorkor results from severe protein deficiency without a calorie deficit. It occurs most commonly in children ages 1 to 3. In the United States, it's usually secondary to:
- malabsorption disorders
- cancer and cancer therapies
- kidney disease
- hypermetabolic illness
- iatrogenic causes.

Marasmus

The third form of malnutrition, marasmus, is a prolonged and gradual wasting of muscle mass and subcutaneous fat. It's caused by inadequate intake of protein, calories, and other nutrients. Marasmus occurs most commonly in infants ages 6 to 18 months, in patients after gastrectomy, and in those with cancer of the mouth and esophagus.

Assessing nutrition

When illness or surgery compromises a patient's intake or alters his metabolic requirements, the relationship between nutrients consumed and energy expended needs to be assessed. A nutritional assessment provides insight into how well the patient's physiologic need for nutrients is being met. Because poor nutritional status can affect most body systems, a thorough nutritional assessment helps anticipate problems and intervene appropriately. To assess nutritional status, these steps are followed:
- A dietary history is obtained.
- A physical assessment is performed.
- Anthropometric measurements are gathered.
- Results of pertinent diagnostic tests are reviewed.

Because poor nutritional status can affect most body systems, a thorough nutritional assessment helps all caregivers anticipate problems and intervene appropriately.

> ### Signs of poor nutrition
>
> When a physical assessment is performed, the patient's overall condition is noted and the skin, mouth, and teeth are inspected. The following are subtle signs of poor nutrition:
> - poor skin turgor
> - bruising
> - abnormal pigmentation
> - darkening of the mouth lining
> - protruding eyes (exophthalmos)
> - neck swelling
> - adventitious breath sounds
> - dental caries
> - ill-fitting dentures
> - signs of infection or irritation in and around the mouth
> - muscle wasting
> - abdominal wasting, masses, and tenderness and an enlarged liver.

DIETARY HISTORY

When a dietary history is obtained, signs of decreased food intake, increased metabolic requirements, or a combination of the two are checked. Also, a dietary recall is done using either a 24-hour recall or diet diary. Factors that affect food intake and changes in appetite are noted. A weight history is also obtained.

PHYSICAL ASSESSMENT

When a physical assessment is performed, the following is included:
- chief complaint
- present illness
- medical history, including previous major illnesses, injuries, hospitalizations, or surgeries
- allergies and history of intolerance to food and medications
- family history, including familial, genetic, or environmental illnesses
- social history, including environmental, psychological, and sociologic factors that may influence nutritional status, such as alcoholism, living alone, or lack of transportation.
- subtle signs of malnutrition. (See *Signs of poor nutrition*.)

Anthropometry

Anthropometry compares the patient's measurements with established standards. (See *Taking anthropometric measurements*.) It's an objective, noninvasive method for measuring overall body size, composition, and specific body parts. Commonly used anthropometric measurements include:
- height
- weight

Assessing nutrition ■ 259

Taking anthropometric measurements

Follow the steps below to measure mid-arm length, triceps skin-fold thickness, and mid-arm muscle circumference.

MID-ARM LENGTH
Locate the midpoint on the patient's upper arm using a nonstretching tape measure, and mark the midpoint with a marking pen.

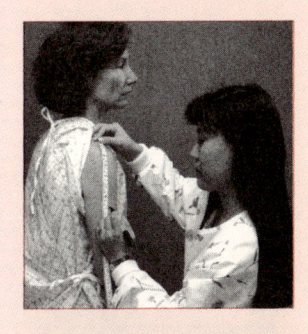

TRICEPS SKIN-FOLD THICKNESS
Determine the triceps skin-fold thickness by grasping the patient's skin between the thumb and forefinger approximately ⅜" (1 cm) above the midpoint. Place the calipers at the midpoint and squeeze the calipers for about 3 seconds. Record the measurement registered on the handle gauge to the nearest 0.5 mm. Take two more readings, and then average all three to compensate for possible error.

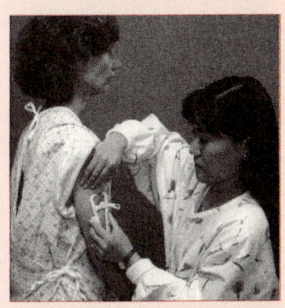

MID-ARM MUSCLE CIRCUMFERENCE
At the midpoint, measure the mid-arm circumference. Calculate the circumference by multiplying the triceps skin-fold thickness (in centimeters) by 3.143 and subtracting the result from the mid-arm circumference.

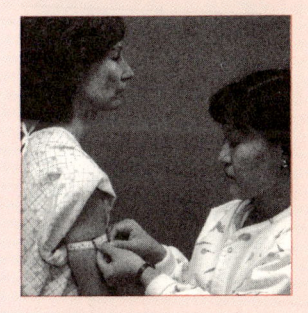

(continued)

> ### Taking anthropometric measurements (continued)
>
> Record all three measurements as percentages of the standard measurements using the following formula:
>
> $$\frac{\text{Actual measurement}}{\text{Standard measurement}} \times 100$$
>
> Compare the patient's percentage measurements with the standard. A measurement of less than 90% of the standard indicates calorie deprivation; a measurement of over 90% of the standard indicates adequate or more than adequate energy reserves.
>
> | MEASUREMENT | STANDARD | 90% |
> |---|---|---|
> | Mid-arm length | Men: 29.3 cm
Women: 26.5 cm | Men: 26.4 cm
Women: 23.9 cm |
> | Triceps skin-fold thickness | Men: 12.5 mm
Women: 16.5 mm | Men: 11.3 mm
Women 14.9 mm |
> | Mid-arm muscle circumference | Men: 25.3 cm
Women 23.2 cm | Men: 22.8 cm
Women: 20.9 cm |

- ideal body weight
- body frame size.

Triceps skin-fold thickness, mid-arm length, and mid-arm muscle circumference are less commonly used anthropometric measurements because they tend to vary by age and race.

A finding of less than 90% of the standard measurement may indicate a need for nutritional support.

DIAGNOSTIC STUDIES

Evidence of a nutritional problem commonly appears in the results of a diagnostic test. Tests are used to evaluate:

- visceral protein status
- lean body mass
- vitamin and mineral balance.

Diagnostic studies are also used to evaluate the effectiveness of nutritional support. (See *Detecting deficiencies*.)

Detecting deficiencies

Laboratory studies help pinpoint nutritional deficiencies by aiding in the diagnosis of anemia, malnutrition, and other disorders. Check out this chart to learn about some commonly ordered diagnostic tests, their purposes, normal values, and implications. Albumin, prealbumin, transferrin, and triglyceride levels are the major indicators of a nutritional deficiency.

TEST AND PURPOSE	NORMAL VALUES	IMPLICATIONS
CREATININE HEIGHT INDEX Uses a 24-hour urine sample to determine adequacy of muscle mass	• Determined from a reference table of values based on a patient's height or weight	• Less than 80% of reference value: moderate depletion of muscle mass (protein reserves) • Less than 60% of reference value: severe depletion, with increased risk of compromised immune function
HEMATOCRIT Diagnoses anemia and dehydration	• Male: 42% to 50% • Female: 40% to 48% • Child: 29% to 41% • Neonate: 55% to 68%	• Increased values: severe dehydration, polycythemia • Decreased values: iron-deficiency anemia, excessive blood loss
HEMOGLOBIN Assesses blood's oxygen-carrying capacity to aid in the diagnosis of anemia, protein deficiency, and hydration status	• Older adult: 10 to 17 g/dl • Adult male: 13 to 18 g/dl • Adult female: 12 to 16 g/dl • Child: 9 to 15.5 g/dl • Neonate: 14 to 20 g/dl	• Increased values: dehydration, polycythemia • Decreased values: protein deficiency, iron-deficiency anemia, excessive blood loss, overhydration
SERUM ALBUMIN Helps assess visceral protein stores	• Adult: 3.5 to 5 g/dl • Child: same as adult • Neonate: 3.6 to 5.4 g/dl	• Decreased values: malnutrition, overhydration, liver or kidney disease, heart failure, excessive blood protein losses such as from severe burns

(continued)

Detecting deficiencies *(continued)*

TEST AND PURPOSE	NORMAL VALUES	IMPLICATIONS
SERUM TRANSFERRIN (similar to serum total iron-binding capacity [TIBC]) Helps assess visceral protein stores; has a shorter half-life than serum albumin and, thus, more accurately reflects current status	• Adult: 200 to 400 mcg/dl • Child: 350 to 450 mcg/dl • Neonate: 60 to 175 mcg/dl	• Increased TIBC: iron deficiency, as in pregnancy or iron deficiency anemia • Decreased TIBC: iron excess, as in chronic inflammatory states • Below 200 mcg/dl: visceral protein depletion • Below 100 mcg/dl: severe visceral protein depletion
SERUM TRIGLYCERIDES Screens for hyperlipidemia	• 40 to 200 mg/dl	• Increased values combined with increased cholesterol levels: increased risk of atherosclerotic disease • Decreased values: protein-energy malnutrition (PEM), steatorrhea
TOTAL LYMPHOCYTE COUNT Diagnoses PEM	• 1,500 to 3,000/µl	• Increased values: infection or inflammation, leukemia, tissue necrosis • Decreased values: moderate to severe malnutrition if no other cause, such as influenza or measles, is identified
TOTAL PROTEIN SCREEN Detects hyperproteinemia or hypoproteinemia	• 6 to 8 g/dl	• Increased values: dehydration • Decreased values: malnutrition, protein loss

Detecting deficiencies *(continued)*

TEST AND PURPOSE	NORMAL VALUES	IMPLICATIONS
TRANSTHYRETIN (PREALBUMIN) Offers information regarding visceral protein stores; should be used in conjunction with albumin level (Prealbumin has a shorter half-life [2 to 3 days] than albumin. This test is sensitive to nutritional repletion.)	• 16 to 40 mg/dl	• Increased values: renal insufficiency; patient on dialysis • Decreased values: PEM, acute catabolic states, postsurgery, hyperthyroidism
URINE KETONE BODIES (ACETONE) Screens for ketonuria and detects carbohydrate deprivation	• Negative for ketones in urine	• Ketoacidosis: starvation

Parenteral nutrition solutions

The solution administered depends on the type of parenteral nutrition and the patient's status. (See *Parenteral solutions,* pages 264 and 265.)

Parenteral nutrition solutions may contain the following elements, each offering a particular benefit:

- Dextrose provides most of the calories that can help maintain nitrogen balance. The number of nonprotein calories needed to maintain nitrogen balance depends on the severity of the patient's illness.
- Amino acids supply enough protein to replace essential amino acids, maintain protein stores, and prevent protein loss from muscle tissues.
- Fats, supplied as lipid emulsions, are a concentrated source of energy that prevent or correct fatty-acid deficiencies. These are available in several concentrations and can provide 30% to 50% of a patient's daily calorie requirement.

Parenteral solutions

THERAPY AND SOLUTIONS	INDICATIONS	SPECIAL CONSIDERATIONS
TOTAL PARENTERAL NUTRITION ● Dextrose, 20% to 70% (1 L dextrose 25% = 850 nonprotein calories) ● Crystalline amino acids, 2.5% to 15% ● Electrolytes, vitamins, micronutrients, insulin, and heparin as ordered ● Fat emulsion, 10% or 20% (can be given peripherally or centrally) ● Water	Long-term therapy (2 weeks or more) is used to: ● supply large quantities of nutrients and calories (2,000 to 3,000 calories per day or more) ● provide needed calories, restore nitrogen balance, replace essential vitamins, electrolytes, minerals, and trace elements ● promote tissue synthesis, wound healing, and normal metabolic function ● allow bowel rest and healing, reduce activity in the pancreas and small intestine ● improve tolerance to surgery if severely malnourished.	● Is nutritionally complete ● Requires surgical procedure for central venous (CV) catheter insertion (can be done by a physician at the patient's bedside) ● May result in metabolic complications (glucose intolerance or electrolyte imbalances) from hypertonic solution ● May not be effective in severely stressed patients (such as those with sepsis or burns) ● May interfere with immune mechanisms

- Electrolytes and minerals are added to the parenteral nutrition solution based on an evaluation of the patient's serum chemistry profile and metabolic needs.
- Vitamins ensure normal body functions and optimal nutrient use. A commercially available mixture of fat- and water-soluble vitamins, biotin, and folic acid may be added to the patient's parenteral nutrition solution.
- Micronutrients, also called *trace elements,* promote normal metabolism. Most commercial solutions contain zinc, copper, chromium, selenium, and manganese.
- Water is added to a parenteral nutrition solution based on the patient's fluid requirements and electrolyte balance.

Parenteral solutions (continued)

THERAPY AND SOLUTIONS

PERIPHERAL PARENTERAL NUTRITION
- Dextrose, 5% to 10%
- Crystalline amino acids, 2.75% to 4.25%
- Electrolytes, minerals, micronutrients, and vitamins as ordered
- Fat emulsion, 10% or 20%
- Heparin or hydrocortisone as ordered
- Water

INDICATIONS

Short-term therapy (3 weeks or less) is used to:
- maintain nutritional state in patients who can tolerate a relatively high fluid volume, who usually resume bowel function and oral feedings in a few days, and who aren't candidates for CV catheters
- provide approximately 1,300 to 1,800 calories per day.

SPECIAL CONSIDERATIONS

- Is nutritionally complete for short-term therapy
- Shouldn't be used in nutritionally depleted patients
- Can't be used in volume-restricted patients because it requires high volumes of solution
- Avoids insertion and maintenance of CV catheter, but the patient must have good veins; I.V. site should be changed every 72 hours
- Delivers less hypertonic solutions
- May cause phlebitis
- Offers a lower risk of metabolic complications

I.V. lipid emulsion
- Has increased risk of hyperlipidemia
- Irritates vein in long-term use

Depending on the patient's condition, a physician may also order additives for the parenteral nutrition solution, such as insulin or heparin. (See *Understanding common additives*, page 266.)

TOTAL PARENTERAL NUTRITION SOLUTIONS

Solutions for total parenteral nutrition (TPN) are hypertonic, with an osmolarity of 1,800 to 2,600 mOsm/L. Electrolytes, minerals, vitamins, micronutrients, and water are added to the base solution to satisfy daily requirements. Lipids may be given as a separate solution or as an admixture with dextrose and amino acids.

Daily allotments of TPN solution, including lipids and other parenteral solution components, are commonly given in a single 3 L

Understanding common additives

Common parenteral nutrition solutions include dextrose 50% in water ($D_{50}W$), amino acids, and any of the additives listed here, which are used to treat the patient's specific metabolic deficiencies:

- Acetate prevents metabolic acidosis.
- Amino acids provide protein necessary for tissue repair.
- Calcium promotes development of bones and teeth and aids in blood clotting.
- Chloride regulates the acid-base equilibrium and maintains osmotic pressure.
- $D_{50}W$ provides calories for metabolism.
- Folic acid is needed for deoxyribonucleic acid formation and promotes growth and development.
- Magnesium aids carbohydrate and protein absorption.
- Micronutrients, such as zinc, manganese, and cobalt, help in wound healing and red blood cell synthesis.
- Phosphate minimizes the potential for developing peripheral paresthesia (numbness and tingling of the extremities).
- Potassium is needed for cellular activity and tissue synthesis.
- Sodium helps regulate water distribution and maintain normal fluid balance.
- Vitamin B complex aids the final absorption of carbohydrates and protein.
- Vitamin C helps in wound healing.
- Vitamin D is essential for bone metabolism and maintenance of the serum calcium level.
- Vitamin K helps prevent bleeding disorders.

---

bag, called a total nutrient admixture, or 3:1 solution. (See *Understanding total nutrient admixture.*)

Glucose balance is extremely important in a patient receiving TPN. Adults use 0.8 to 1 g of glucose per kilogram of body weight per hour. That means a patient can tolerate a constant I.V. infusion of hyperosmolar (highly concentrated) glucose without adding insulin to the solution. As the concentrated glucose solution infuses, a pancreatic beta-cell response causes serum insulin levels to increase.

To allow the pancreas to establish and maintain the necessary increased insulin production, start with a slow infusion rate and increase it gradually as ordered. Abruptly stopping the infusion may cause rebound hypoglycemia, which calls for an infusion of dextrose.

Glucose balance may be further thrown off by:
- sepsis
- stress

> ## Understanding total nutrient admixture
>
> Total nutrient admixture is a white solution that delivers 1 day's worth of nutrients in a single 3-L bag. Also called *3:1 solution*, it combines lipids with other parenteral solution components.
>
> **ADVANTAGES**
> The advtantages of total nutrient admixture include:
> - less need to handle the bag (lower risk of contamination)
> - less time required
> - less need for infusion sets and electronic infusion devices
> - lower hospital costs
> - increased patient mobility
> - easier adjustment to home care.
>
> **DISADVANTAGES**
> The disadvantages of total nutrient admixture include:
> - use of certain infusion devices precluded because of their inability to accurately deliver large volumes of solution
> - 1.2-micron filter required (rather than a 0.22-micron filter) to allow lipid molecules through
> - limited amount of calcium and phosphorus added because of the difficulty in detecting precipitate in the milky white solution.

- shock
- liver or kidney failure
- diabetes
- age
- pancreatic disease
- use of certain medications, including steroids.

PERIPHERAL PARENTERAL SOLUTIONS

Peripheral parenteral nutrition (PPN) solutions usually consist of dextrose 5% in water to 10% dextrose and 2.75% to 4.25% crystalline amino acids. Or, PPN solutions may be slightly hypertonic, such as dextrose 10% in water, with an osmolarity no greater than 600 mOsm/L. Lipid emulsions, electrolytes, trace elements, and vitamins may be given as part of PPN to add calories and other needed nutrients.

Lipid emulsions

In an oral diet, lipids or fats are the major source of calories, usually providing about 40% of the total calorie intake. In parenteral nutrition solutions, lipids provide 9 kcal/g. I.V. lipid emulsions are oxidized for energy as needed. As a nearly isotonic emulsion, concentrations of 10% or 20% can be safely infused through peripheral or central veins. Lipid emulsions prevent and treat essential fatty acid deficiency and provide a major source of energy.

Giving parenteral nutrition

Parenteral nutrition is delivered in one of two ways: continuously or cyclically. With continuous delivery, the patient receives the infusion over a 24-hour period. The infusion begins at a slow rate and increases to the optional rate as ordered. This type of delivery may prevent complications, such as hyperglycemia, from a high dextrose load.

A patient undergoing cyclic therapy receives the entire 24-hour volume of parenteral nutrition solution over a shorter period, perhaps 10, 12, 14, or 16 hours. Home care parenteral nutrition programs have boosted the use of cyclic therapy. This type of therapy may be used to wean the patient from total parenteral nutrition (TPN). (See *Switching from continuous to cyclic TPN.*)

GIVING TOTAL PARENTERAL NUTRITION

Administering TPN doesn't fall under the scope of practice for the LPN, but it's important to know about the methods so you can help support the patient throughout the process.

TPN solutions must be infused in a central vein, using one of the following methods:
- a peripherally inserted catheter (with its tip lying in a central vein)
- a central venous (CV) catheter
- an implanted infusion device.

Long-term therapy requires use of one of the following:
- a Silastic CV catheter, such as a Hickman, Broviac, or Groshong catheter
- an implanted reservoir such as an Infus-A-Port
- an implanted infusion device.

Because TPN fluid has about six times the solute concentration of blood, peripheral I.V. administration can cause sclerosis and thrombosis. To ensure adequate dilution, the CV catheter is inserted into the superior vena cava, a wide-bore, high-flow vein. Usually, the catheter isn't advanced into the right atrium because of the risk of cardiac perforation and arrhythmias.

> **BEST PRACTICE**
> ## Switching from continuous to cyclic TPN
>
> When switching from continuous to cyclic total parenteral nutrition (TPN), the infusion rate is adjusted so the patient's blood glucose level can adapt to the decreased nutrient load. This is done by reducing the infusion rate by one-half for 1 hour before stopping the infusion. A blood glucose sample is drawn 1 hour after the infusion ends, and the patient is observed for signs of hypoglycemia, such as sweating, shakiness, and irritability.

Preparing the patient

To increase compliance, you can assist in preparing the patient by making sure that he understands the purpose of treatment and by enlisting his help throughout the course of therapy.

Understanding TPN and its goals helps a home care patient assume a greater role in administering, monitoring, and maintaining therapy. When instructing a home care patient, teaching focuses on signs and symptoms of:
- fluid, electrolyte, or glucose imbalance
- vitamin and trace element deficiencies and toxicities
- catheter infection, such as fever, chills, discomfort on infusion, and redness or drainage at the catheter insertion site.

To help prevent glucose imbalance, the patient receiving his first I.V. bag of TPN should be taught how to regulate the infusion rate so he can maintain the rate prescribed by the physician. It should be explained that a gradual increase in the infusion rate allows the pancreas to establish and maintain the increased insulin production necessary to tolerate this treatment. When the goal rate of the TPN infusion is met, the rate shouldn't need to be adjusted.

Finally, the details of the administration schedule, the equipment the patient will use, how to avoid incompatibility, and the prescribed and over-the-counter medications he takes should all be reviewed with the patient.

To safely maintain this therapy, the prescribed regimen must be adhered to by the patient and his caregivers. Your teaching efforts and return demonstrations by the patient help to boost compliance in all aspects of TPN therapy.

> **BEST PRACTICE**
>
> ## Administering lipid emulsions
>
> Most total parenteral nutrition solutions contain lipid emulsions. To safely administer them, follow these special precautions:
>
> ● Monitor the patient's vital signs and watch for adverse reactions, such as fever, a pressure sensation over the eyes, nausea, vomiting, headache, chest and back pain, tachycardia, dyspnea, cyanosis, and flushing, sweating, or chills. If the patient has no adverse reactions to the test dose, the infusion can begin at the prescribed rate.
>
> ● Before the infusion, the parenteral nutrition with lipids should be checked for separation or an oily appearance. If either condition exists, the lipid may have come out of emulsion and shouldn't be used.
>
> ● Because lipid emulsions are at high risk for bacterial growth, a partially empty bottle of emulsion should never be rehung.

Preparing the equipment

Before TPN administration begins, the physician inserts an infusion device. The device may be a CV catheter or an implanted device. The location of the catheter tip is confirmed by X-ray.

Then the following equipment is gathered: the TPN solution, a pump, an administration set with a filter, alcohol swabs, gloves, and an I.V. pole. Hands should be washed before preparing the TPN solution for administration, and the administration set should be prepared in a clean area.

Tubing with a filter is always used when administering TPN. Filters are required by the Food and Drug Administration.

The infusion of a chilled solution can cause discomfort, hypothermia, venous spasm, and venous constriction. The bag or bottle of TPN solution should be removed from the refrigerator about 30 minutes before hanging it to allow for warming.

Checking the order

The written order is checked against the label on the bag to make sure that the volumes, concentrations, and additives are included in the solution and that the infusion rate is correct. The patient's identity should be confirmed using two patient identifiers (neither being the patient's room number).

RED FLAG Careful inspection of the infusate should be a habit. It should be checked for clouding, floating debris, or a change in color. Any of these phenomena could indicate contam-

Giving parenteral nutrition ■ 271

> **BEST PRACTICE**
> ## Reducing the risk of infection
>
> Because a total parenteral nutrition (TPN) solution serves as a medium for bacterial growth and a central venous line provides systemic access, the patient receiving TPN risks infection and sepsis. According to the Centers for Disease Control and Prevention, maintaining strict aseptic technique when handling the equipment used to administer therapy has been shown to reduce the number of TPN-related infections.

ination, problems with the integrity of the solution, or a pH change. If you see anything suspicious, the pharmacy should be notified.

The physician will be informed that there may be a delay in hanging the solution and he may want to order dextrose 10% in water until a new container of TPN solution is available. Also, the solution will be returned to the pharmacy.

Most TPN solutions contain lipid emulsions, which call for special precautions. (See *Administering lipid emulsions*.)

Beginning the infusion

RED FLAG *When the infusion is started, the catheter insertion site should be checked for swelling. This may indicate extravasation of the TPN solution, which can cause necrosis (tissue damage).* (See Reducing the risk of infection.)

Maintaining the infusion

If the patient tolerates the solution well the first day, the physician usually increases intake to the goal rate by the second day. To maintain a TPN infusion, these key steps are followed:

RED FLAG *When using a single-lumen CV catheter, the line shouldn't be used to piggyback or infuse blood or blood products, give a bolus injection, administer simultaneous I.V. solutions, measure CV pressure, or draw blood for laboratory tests. In unavoidable circumstances, the TPN port may be used for electrolyte replacement or insulin drips. Drugs should never be added to the container. Also, using add-on devices should be avoided because they increase the risk of infection.*

- The order is checked against the label on the TPN container.
- The container is labeled with the expiration date, time at which the solution was hung, glucose concentration, and total volume of solution.

Precautions when maintaining a TPN infusion

- If the bag or bottle is damaged and an immediate replacement isn't available, the glucose concentration can be approximated until a new container is ready by adding 50% glucose to dextrose 10% in water.
- All tubing junctions are secured tightly.
- Gravity should never be used to administer total parenteral nutrition (TPN).
- Stay alert for increased body temperature — one of the earliest signs of catheter-related sepsis.
- Typically, alanine aminotransferase, aspartate aminotransferase, alkaline phosphatase, cholesterol, triglyceride, plasma-free fatty acid, and coagulation tests are performed weekly.
- A patient may require supplementary insulin throughout TPN therapy; the pharmacy usually adds insulin directly to the TPN solution.
- If the dressing becomes wet, soiled, or nonocclusive, it can be changed more frequently than every 48 hours.
- Report abnormal laboratory test results to the physician so that he can adjust the TPN solution appropriately.

- Infusion rates are maintained as prescribed, even if the infusion falls behind schedule.
- TPN solutions shouldn't hang for more than 24 hours.
- The tubing and filter are changed every 24 hours, using strict aseptic technique.
- I.V. site care and dressing changes are performed according to the facility's policy and protocol—usually every 48 hours.
- The infusion pump's volume meter and time tape are checked every 30 minutes (or more often, if necessary) to monitor for irregular flow rate.
- Vital signs are recorded when therapy is initiated and every 4 to 8 hours thereafter (or more often, if necessary).
- The patient's glucose levels should be monitored as ordered using glucose fingersticks or serum tests.
- The patient's daily fluid intake and output should be recorded specifying the volume and type of each fluid to assure prompt, precise replacement of fluid and electrolytes.
- The patient should be weighed at the same time each morning (after voiding), in similar clothing, using the same scale. Suspect fluid imbalance if the patient gains more than 1 lb (0.5 kg) per day. Anthropometric measurements may be ordered.

Giving parenteral nutrition ■ 273

- Routine laboratory tests, such as electrolyte, blood urea nitrogen, and glucose levels, are monitored, and abnormal findings are reported to the physician.
- The triglyceride level, which should be in the normal range during continuous TPN infusion, is checked.
- The patient should be monitored for signs and symptoms of nutritional aberrations, such as fluid and electrolyte imbalance or glucose metabolism disturbance.
- Patients commonly associate eating with positive feelings and become disturbed when it's eliminated. Emotional support should be provided.
- Frequent mouth care should be provided for the patient.
- All assessment findings and nursing interventions should be documented.
- Take the needed precautions. (See *Precautions when maintaining a TPN infusion*.)

GIVING PERIPHERAL PARENTERAL NUTRITION

Using an amino acid, dextrose, and lipid emulsion solution, peripheral parenteral nutrition (PPN) fulfills a patient's basic calorie needs without the risks involved in CV access. Because PPN solutions have lower tonicity than TPN solutions, a patient receiving PPN must be able to tolerate the infusion of large volumes of fluid. PPN is administered through a peripheral vein, but doesn't usually fall under the scope of practice for LPNs. Check your state's nurse practice act for details.

Preparing the patient

You can help prepare the patient by making sure that he understands what to expect before, during, and after therapy.

The patient's largest available vein is selected as the insertion site. This enables blood to adequately dilute the PPN solution, which can be irritating. When using a short-term catheter, the site is rotated every 48 to 72 hours, or according to facility policy and procedures.

Preparing the equipment

To administer PPN, the necessary equipment needs to be gathered, including:
- ordered PPN solution (at room temperature)
- infusion pump
- administration set
- alcohol swabs

- I.V. pole
- venipuncture equipment, if needed.

Checking the order
The written order is checked against the written label on the bag. The solution should be for peripheral infusion, and the volumes, concentrations, and additives should be included in the solution. The infusion rate is also checked. The patient's identity should be confirmed using two patient identifiers (neither being the patient's room number).

In PPN therapy, lipid emulsions may be part of the solution. If given separately, the lipid emulsion is piggybacked below the in-line filter close to the insertion site. This prevents the possibility of lipids clogging the filtration system. When giving lipids, controllers that can accommodate lipid emulsions should be used.

Beginning the infusion
***RED FLAG** When the PPN infusion is started as ordered, the peripheral insertion site should be checked for swelling. Swelling may indicate infiltration or extravasation of the PPN solution, which can cause tissue damage.*

Maintaining the infusion
Caring for a patient receiving a PPN infusion involves the same steps required for any patient receiving a peripheral I.V. infusion. The infusion rate needs to be maintained and the tubing, dressings, infusion site, and I.V. devices need to be cared for.

***RED FLAG** Sepsis, the most serious catheter-related complication, can be fatal. This can be prevented by meticulous, consistent catheter care. If the patient is developing catheter-related sepsis, he may develop an unexplained fever, chills, and a red, indurated area around the catheter site. The patient may also have unexplained hyperglycemia, commonly an early warning sign of sepsis. (See Monitoring for signs and symptoms of sepsis.)*

Because the synthesis of lipase (a fat-splitting enzyme) increases insulin requirements, the insulin dosage of a patient with diabetes may need to be increased. Insulin is one of the additives that may be adjusted in the formulation of the PPN solution.

For a patient with hypothyroidism, thyroid-stimulating hormone (TSH) may need to be administered. TSH affects lipase activity and may prevent triglycerides from accumulating in the vascular system.

Monitoring for signs and symptoms of sepsis

The patient should be monitored for signs or symptoms of sepsis, including:
- elevated temperature
- glucose in urine (glycosuria)
- chills
- malaise
- increased white blood cells (leukocytosis)
- altered level of consciousness
- elevated glucose levels, measured by fingerstick or serum chemistry.

Patients receiving lipid emulsions commonly report a feeling of fullness or bloating; occasionally, they experience an unpleasant metallic or greasy taste. A patient may develop an allergic reaction to the fat emulsion.

Early adverse reactions to lipid emulsion therapy occur in less than 1% of patients. These reactions may include:
- fever
- difficulty breathing
- cyanosis
- nausea
- vomiting
- headache
- flushing
- sweating
- lethargy
- dizziness
- chest and back pain
- slight pressure over the eyes
- irritation at the infusion site.

Changes in laboratory test results may also reveal problems when a patient receives lipid emulsions, including:
- hyperlipidemia
- hypercoagulability
- thrombocytopenia.

The physician monitors the patient's lipid emulsion clearance rate. The lipid emulsion may clear from the blood at an accelerated rate in a patient with severe burns, multiple trauma, or a metabolic imbalance.

Stopping therapy

One major difference exists between the procedures for discontinuing total parenteral nutrition (TPN) and peripheral parenteral nutrition (PPN) therapy. A patient receiving TPN should be weaned from therapy and should receive some other form of nutritional therapy such as enteral feedings.

When the patient is receiving PPN, therapy can be stopped without weaning because the dextrose concentration is lower than in TPN. When stopping TPN therapy, the patient should be weaned over 24 hours to prevent rebound hypoglycemia.

Precautions and complications

LIFE STAGES *Pediatric and elderly patients are particularly susceptible to fluid overload and heart failure. With these patients, it's important to administer the correct volume of parenteral nutrition solution at the correct infusion rate.*

CHILDREN
Parenteral feeding therapy for children serves a dual purpose.
- It maintains a child's nutritional status.
- It fuels a child's growth.

Children have a greater need than adults for certain nutrients. This is an important consideration in accurately calculating solution components for children. Overall, children have a greater need than adults for nutrients, including:
- protein
- carbohydrates
- fat
- electrolytes
- micronutrients
- vitamins
- fluids.

As with adults, children receiving total parenteral nutrition (TPN) should be evaluated carefully by the nurse, physician, and nutritional support team. The following factors are considered when planning to meet children's nutritional needs:
- age
- weight
- activity level
- size

- development
- calorie needs.

Administering peripheral parenteral nutrition (PPN) with lipid emulsions in a premature or low-birth-weight infant may lead to lipid accumulation in the lungs. Thrombocytopenia (platelet deficiency) has also been reported in infants receiving 20% lipid emulsions.

ELDERLY PATIENTS

RED FLAG In an elderly patient, overinfusion can produce serious adverse effects, so always monitor flow rates carefully. The elderly patient is also at risk for fluid overload when TPN or PPN is given.

An elderly patient may have underlying clinical problems that affect the treatment outcome. For example, he may be taking medications that interact with the components in the parenteral nutrition solution. For this reason, the pharmacist should be consulted about possible interactions.

COMPLICATIONS

A patient receiving parenteral nutrition therapy faces many of the same complications as a patient undergoing any type of peripheral I.V. or central venous (CV) therapy. (See *Handling TPN hazards*, pages 278 and 279.)

Complications of parenteral nutrition therapy may result from problems that are:
- catheter-related
- metabolic
- mechanical.

Catheter-related complications

The most common catheter-related complications include:
- clotting
- dislodgment
- cracked or broken tubing
- pneumothorax and hydrothorax
- sepsis.

Suspect a clotted catheter if the infusion rate is interrupted. You may also notice that a greater pressure is needed to maintain the infusion at the desired rate.

When the catheter comes out of the vein, catheter dislodgment may be obvious. You may note that the dressing is wet. The patient may report feeling cold or that his gown is wet. When the catheter

Handling TPN hazards

Complications of total parenteral nutrition (TPN) can result from catheter-related, metabolic, or mechanical problems. To find out how these complications are treated, use this chart.

COMPLICATIONS	INTERVENTIONS
CATHETER-RELATED COMPLICATIONS	
Clotted catheter	● The catheter is repositioned. ● Alteplase (tPA) is instilled to clear the catheter lumen as ordered.
Dislodged catheter	● A sterile gauze pad treated with antimicrobial ointment is placed on the insertion site, and pressure applied.
Cracked or broken tubing	● A padded hemostat is applied above the break to prevent air from entering the line.
Pneumothorax	● A chest tube is inserted. ● Chest tube suctioning is maintained as ordered.
Sepsis	● The catheter is removed and the tip is cultured. ● Appropriate antibiotics are given.
METABOLIC COMPLICATIONS	
Hyperglycemia	● Insulin therapy is started or the TPN flow rate is adjusted as ordered.
Hypoglycemia	● Dextrose is infused as ordered.
Hyperosmolar hyperglycemic nonketotic syndrome	● Dextrose is stopped. ● The patient is rehydrated with the ordered infusate.
Hypokalemia	● Potassium supplementation is increased.
Hypomagnesemia	● Magnesium supplementation is increased.
Hypophosphatemia	● Phosphate supplementation is increased.
Hypocalcemia	● Calcium supplementation is increased.

Handling TPN hazards *(continued)*

COMPLICATIONS	INTERVENTIONS
METABOLIC COMPLICATIONS *(continued)*	
Metabolic acidosis	• The formula is adjusted and the patient is assessed for contributing factors.
Liver dysfunction	• Carbohydrates are decreased and I.V. lipids are added. • Cyclic infusions are considered.
Hyperkalemia	• Potassium supplementation is decreased.
MECHANICAL COMPLICATIONS	
Air embolism	• The catheter is clamped. • The patient is placed in Trendelenburg's position on the left side. • Oxygen is given as ordered. • If cardiac arrest occurs, cardiopulmonary resuscitation is initiated.
Venous thrombosis	• The physician is notified. • Heparin is administered, if ordered. • Venous flow studies may be done.
Too rapid an infusion	• The infusion rate is checked. • The infusion pump is checked.
Extravasation	• The I.V. infusion is stopped. • The patient is assessed for cardiopulmonary abnormalities. Chest X-ray may be performed.
Phlebitis	• Gentle heat is applied to the insertion site. • The insertion site is elevated, if possible.

is located peripherally, the area around the insertion site may be red or swollen from subcutaneous extravasation of the PPN solution. With a centrally inserted catheter, there may be swelling and redness around the insertion site. The most significant complications include bleeding from the insertion site or an air embolism.

If the catheter or vascular access device is damaged, infusate may leak from a cracked area or the insertion site. If the infusion tubing is damaged, the I.V. insertion site remains dry. Both situations require immediate attention because of the risk of bleeding, contamination, or air emboli.

Pneumothorax usually results from trauma to the pleura during insertion of a CV access device. The patient may have dyspnea and chest pain; he may also develop a cough. Auscultation reveals diminished breath sounds, and the patient may be sweating and appear cyanotic. Assessment may also reveal unilateral chest movement. Pneumothorax should be confirmed by X-ray for the best treatment results.

Metabolic complications

Metabolic complications include:
- hyperglycemia or hypoglycemia
- hyperkalemia or hypokalemia
- hypomagnesemia
- hypophosphatemia
- hypocalcemia.

See *Understanding metabolic complications* for a complete description of each of these.

Mechanical complications

Mechanical complications that can plague parenteral nutrition therapy include:
- air embolism
- venous thrombosis
- extravasation
- phlebitis.

RED FLAG *Suspect an air embolism if the patient develops apprehension, chest pain, tachycardia, hypotension, cyanosis, seizures, loss of consciousness, or cardiac arrest. Auscultation may also reveal the classic sign of an air embolism—a churning heart murmur.*

RED FLAG *Suspect thrombosis when you see redness or swelling at the catheter insertion site or swelling of the arm, neck, or face. Other signs and symptoms include pain at the insertion site and along the vein, malaise, fever, and tachycardia.*

If TPN is infused too rapidly, the patient may feel nauseated, have a headache, and become lethargic. Heart failure is also a risk from fluid overload. If you observe swelling of the tissue around the insertion site, it may indicate extravasation. The patient may also complain of pain at the insertion site. Pain, tenderness, redness, and warmth at the insertion site and along the vein path may indicate phlebitis.

Understanding metabolic complications

COMPLICATION	POSSIBLE CAUSES	SIGNS AND SYMPTOMS
Hyperglycemia	• Glucose concentration is excessive • Infusion rate too rapid • Diabetes • Stress • Sepsis	• Fatigue • Restlessness • Weakness • Anxiety • Confusion, leading to delirium • Dehydration • Polyuria • If left untreated, hyperosmolar hyperglycemic nonketotic syndrome, (HHNS) characterized by lethargy, seizures, high serum osmolarity, and extremely high glucose level – as high as 600 to 4,800 mg/dl • If HHNS goes untreated, glycosuria, electrolyte disturbances, and eventually coma
Hypoglycemia	• Parenteral nutrition interrupted suddenly • Excessive insulin	• Sweating • Shaking • Confusion • Irritability
Hyperkalemia	• Too much potassium in solution • Renal disease • Hyponatremia	• Skeletal-muscle weakness • Decreased heart rate • Irregular pulse • Tall T waves on the ECG strip
Hypokalemia	• Too little potassium in solution • GI tract disturbances • Diuretic use • Large doses of insulin	• Muscle weakness • Paralysis • Paresthesia • Cardiac arrhythmias

(continued)

Understanding metabolic complications (*continued*)

COMPLICATION	POSSIBLE CAUSES	SIGNS AND SYMPTOMS
Hypomagnesemia	• Too little magnesium in solution	• Tingling around the mouth • Paresthesia in the fingers • Mental changes • Hyperreflexia • Tetany • Arrhythmia
Hypophosphatemia	• Insulin therapy • Alcoholism • Use of phosphate-binding antacids	• Irritability • Weakness • Paresthesia • Coma and cardiac arrest (in extreme cases)
Hypocalcemia (rare)	• Too little calcium in the solution • Vitamin D deficiency • Pancreatitis	• Numbness or tingling • Tetany • Polyuria • Dehydration • Arrhythmia

Complications of peripheral parenteral nutrition and lipid emulsions

PPN and lipid emulsion administration pose distinct risks. Significant complications of PPN therapy include phlebitis, infiltration, and extravasation.

Prolonged administration of lipid emulsions can produce delayed complications, including an enlarged liver or spleen, blood dyscrasia (thrombocytopenia and leukopenia), and transient increases in the results of liver function studies. A small number of patients receiving 20% I.V. lipid emulsion develop brown pigmentation from fat pigmentation.

Dangerous abbreviations

Using a flow sheet to document I.V therapy

Common fluid and electrolyte imbalances in children

Common fluid and electrolyte imbalances in eldery patients

Selected references

Index

Dangerous abbreviations

The Joint Commission on Accreditation of Healthcare Organizations has agreed upon a list of dangerous abbreviations, acronyms, and symbols. Using this list should help protect patients from the effects of miscommunication in clinical documentation.

ABBREVIATION	DANGER	PREFERRED USE
U or u (for "unit")	Mistaken for the numbers 0 or 4 (for example, 4U seen as 40 or 4u seen as 44). Also mistaken for "cc" (for example, 4u seen as 4cc).	Write "unit."
IU (for "international unit")	Mistaken for I.V. (intravenous) or 10 (ten).	Write "international unit."
q.d. (Latin abbreviation for "every day")	Mistaken for q.i.d., especially if the period after the "q" or the tail of the "q" could be seen as an "i."	Write "daily" or "once daily."
q.o.d. (Latin abbreviation "every other day")	Mistaken for q.d. or q.i.d. if the "o" is poorly written.	Write "every other day."
Trailing zero (such as 1.0 mg)	Decimal point may be missed (for example, 1.0 may be seen as 10).	Never write a zero by itself after a decimal point (1 mg rather than 1.0 mg).
Lack of leading zero (such as .5 mg)	Decimal point may be missed (for example, .5 may be seen as 5).	Always write a zero before a decimal point (0.5 mg rather than .5 mg).
MS or MSO$_4$ (morphine sulfate)	Mistaken for magnesium sulfate.	Write "morphine sulfate."
MgSO$_4$ (magnesium sulfate)	Mistaken for morphine sulfate.	Write "magnesium sulfate."

©Joint Commission on Accreditation of Healthcare Organizations, 2005. Reprinted with permission.

Using a flow sheet to document I.V. therapy

The sample below shows the typical features of an I.V. therapy flow sheet.

I.V. Therapy Flow Sheet

Patient: James Tolman
Diagnosis: ℞ total hip replacement
Venipuncture limitations ℞ arm only
Permanent access: None

INTRAVENOUS CARE COMMENT CODES C = CAP F = FILTER T= TUBING D = DRESSING									
START DATE/ TIME	INITIALS	I.V. VOLUME & SOLUTION	ADDITIVES	FLOW RATE	SITE	STOP DATE/ TIME	CHANGE	COMMENTS
6/30/06 1100	DS	1000 cc D_5W	20 meq KCL	100/hr	RFA	6/30/06 2100	T	
6/30/06 2100	JM	1000 cc D_5W	20 meq KCL	100/hr	RFA	7/1/06 0700		
7/1/06 0700	DS	1000 cc D_5W	20 meq KCL	100/hr	7/2/05 LFA		TD	

Common fluid and electrolyte imbalances in children

Imbalance	Causes	Signs and symptoms	Treatment
Hyperkalemia (serum potassium > 5 mEq/L [> 5 mmol/L])	• Acute acidosis • Addison's disease • Excessive administration of I.V. potassium supplement • Hemolysis or rhabdomyolysis • Renal failure	• Arrhythmia • Dry, sticky mucous membranes • Electrocardiogram (ECG) changes (tall, tented T waves; ST-segment depression; prolonged PR interval and QRS complex; and absent P waves) • Flushed skin • Hoarsenesss • Intense thirst • Nausea • Paresthesia • Vomiting • Weakness	• Bicarbonate (for acidosis) • Dialysis (for renal failure) • I.V. calcium gluconate (antagonizes cardiac abnormalities) • I.V. insulin or hypertonic dextrose solution (shifts potassium into the cells) • Restricted potassium intake • Sodium polystyrene (Kayexalate) (to remove potassium via the GI tract)
Hypokalemia (serum potassium < 3.5 mEq/L [< 3.5 mmol/L])	• Acute alkalosis • Diarrhea • Diuretic use • Kidney disease • Malabsorption • Nasogastric suctioning • Starvation • Vomiting	• Apathy • Decreased bowel motility • Drowsiness • ECG changes (flattened or inverted T waves, presence of U waves, and ST-segment depression) • Fatigue • Hyporeflexia • Hypotension • Irritability • Muscle cramping	• Oral or I.V. potassium administration (I.V. infusions must be diluted and given slowly)

Imbalance	Causes	Signs and Symptoms	Treatment
Hypokalemia *(continued)*		• Muscle weakness • Paralysis • Tachycardia or bradycardia	
Hypernatremia (serum sodium > 145 mEq/L [> 145 mmol/L])	• Diabetes insipidus (insufficient antidiuretic hormone [ADH] production or reduced response to ADH) • Diarrhea • Fever • Hyperglycemia • Insufficient water intake • Renal disease • Vomiting • Water loss in excess of sodium loss	• Confusion • Decreased blood pressure • Decreased skin turgor • Dry, sticky mucous membranes • Flushed skin • Intense thirst • Hoarseness • Nausea • Seizures • Tachycardia • Vomiting	• Gradual replacement of water (in excess of sodium) or ADH replacement or vasopressin administration (for patients with diabetes insipidus)
Hyponatremia (serum sodium < 138 mEq/L [< 138 mmol/L])	• Cystic fibrosis • Edema (from heart failure) • Excess sweating • Fever • Hypotonic fluid replacement (for diarrhea) • Malnutrition • Syndrome of inappropriate antidiuretic hormone	• Abdominal cramps • Apprehension • Dehydration • Dizziness • Nausea	• Diuretic administration • Fluid replacement (with ongoing fluid loss such as with diarrhea) • Sodium replacement • Water restriction

Common fluid and electrolyte imbalances in children

Imbalance	Causes	Signs and symptoms	Treatment
Hypovolemia (fluid volume deficit)	● Decreased oral intake ● Dehydration ● Diarrhea ● Excessive fluid loss ● Vomiting	● Altered level of consciousness ● Decreased tears ● Depressed fontanels (in infants) ● Dry mucous membranes ● Oliguria or anuria ● Sunken eyes ● Tachycardia ● Thirst ● Weight loss	● Oral rehydration (in mild to moderate dehydration) ● I.V. fluid administration (in severe dehydration) ● Electrolyte replacement

Common fluid and electrolyte imbalances in elderly patients

IMBALANCE	CAUSES	SIGNS AND SYMPTOMS	TREATMENT
Hyperkalemia (serum potassium > 5 mEq/L [> 5 mmol/L])	• Diabetic ketoacidosis • Impaired tubular function • Metabolic acidosis • Potassium-conserving diuretic use (in patients with renal insufficiency) • Rapid I.V. potassium administration • Renal failure	• Arrhythmia • Electrocardiogram (ECG) changes (tall, tented T waves; ST-segment depression; prolonged PR interval and QRS complex; shortened QT interval, absent P waves) • Paresthesia • Weakness	• Bicarbonate (for patients with acidosis) • Dialysis (for patients with renal failure) • I.V. calcium gluconate (antagonizes cardiac abnormalities) • I.V. insulin or hypertonic dextrose solution (shifts potassium into the cells) • Potassium intake restriction • Sodium polystyrene (Kayexalate) (to remove potassium via the GI tract)
Hypokalemia (serum potassium < 3.5 mEq/L [< 3.5 mmol/L])	• Diarrhea • Digoxin toxicity • Diuretic use • Decreased potassium intake • Nasogastric suctioning • Vomiting	• Confusion • Decreased bowel motility • ECG changes (flattened T waves, presence of U waves, and ST-segment depression) • Fatigue • Muscle cramps • Ventricular tachycardia or fibrillation • Weakness • Coma	• Oral or I.V. potassium administration (I.V. infusions must be diluted and given slowly)

Common fluid and electrolyte imbalances in the elderly

Imbalance	Causes	Signs and Symptoms	Treatment
Hypernatremia (serum sodium > 145 mEq/L [> 145 mmol/L])	• Diarrhea • Hypertonic tube feedings without adequate water replacement • Low body weight • Water deprivation	• Dry, mucous membranes • Hallucinations • Hyperreflexia • Irritability • Lethargy • Restlessness • Seizures • Weakness	• Gradual infusion of hypotonic electrolyte solution or isotonic saline solution
Hyponatremia (serum sodium < 138 mEq/L [< 138 mmol/L])	• Diuretics • Excessive I.V. fluids or parenteral feedings • Excessive water intake • Kidney disease • Loss of GI fluids	• Confusion • Coma • Delirium • Diarrhea • Lethargy • Muscle cramps • Nausea and vomiting • Seizures • Weakness	• Gradual sodium replacement, water restriction (1 to 1½ qt [1 to 1.5 L]/day, or discontinuation of diuretuc therapy (if ordered)
Hypervolemia (fluid volume excess)	• Cirrhosis • Coma • Heart failure • Increased oral or I.V. sodium intake • Mental confusion • Renal failure • Seizures	• Bounding pulse • Crackles • Edema • Elevated blood pressure • Increased central venous perssure • Jugular vein distention • Shortness of breath • Weight gain	• Diuretics, fluid restriction (< 1 qt [1 L]/day), sodium restriction, or hemodialysis (for patients with renal failure)

Common fluid and electrolyte imbalances in the elderly

Imbalance	Causes	Signs and Symptoms	Treatment
Hypovolemia (fluid volume deficit)	• Chronic kidney disease • Decreased oral inatke secondary to anorexia • Dehydration • Diabetes mellitus • Diarrhea • Diminished thirst mechanism • Diuretic use • Fever • Hot weather • Inadequate water intake (common in nursing home patients) • Nausea • Polyuria • Vomiting	• Anuria • Confusion or altered mental status • Dizziness • Dry mucous membranes • Increased hemoglobin, hematocrit, blood urea nitrogen, and serum creatinine levels • Oliguria or concentrated urine • Orthostatic hypotension • Possible severe hypotension • Weakness	• Fluid administration (may be oral or I.V. depending on degree of deficit and patient's response; a urine output of 30 to 50 ml/hour usually signals adequate renal perfusion)

Selected references

Alexander, M., and Corrigan, A.M. *Core Curriculum for Infusion Nursing,* 3rd ed. Philadelphia: Lippincott Williams & Wilkins, 2003.

Braunwald, E., et al. *Harrison's Principles of Internal Medicine,* 16th ed. New York: McGraw-Hill Book Co., 2005.

Critical Care Challenges: Disorders, Treatments, and Procedures. Philadelphia: Lippincott Williams & Wilkins, 2003.

Critical Care Nursing Made Incredibly Easy. Philadelphia: Lippincott Williams & Wilkins, 2003.

Fiaccadori, E., et al. "Enteral Nutrition in Patients with Acute Renal Failure," *Kidney International* 65(3):999-1008, March 2004.

Gorski, L.A. "Central Venous Access Device Occlusions: Part 1: Nonthrombotic Causes and Treatment," *Home Healthcare Nurse* 21(2):115-21, February 2003.

Gorski, L.A. "Central Venous Access Device Occlusions: Part 2: Nonthrombotic Causes and Treatment," *Home Healthcare Nurse* 21(3):168-71, March 2003.

Hadaway, L.C. "Infusing Without Infecting," *Nursing2003* 33(10):58-63, October 2003.

I.V. Therapy Made Incredibly Easy, 3rd ed. Philadelphia: Lippincott Williams & Wilkins, 2006.

Ignatavicius, D.D., and Workman, M.L. *Medical-Surgical Nursing Critical Thinking for Collaborative Care,* 4th ed. Philadelphia: W.B. Saunders Co., 2002.

Infusion Nurses Society. *Infusion Therapy in Clinical Practice,* 2nd ed. Philadelphia: W.B. Saunders Co., 2001.

Mims, B.C., et al. *Critical Care Skills: A Clinical Handbook,* 2nd ed. Philadelphia: W.B. Saunders Co., 2004.

Nursing 2006 Drug Handbook, 26th ed. Philadelphia: Lippincott Williams & Wilkins, 2006.

Nursing Procedures, 4th ed. Philadelphia: Lippincott Williams & Wilkins, 2004.

Plummer's Principles & Practice of Intravenous Therapy, 7th ed. Philadelphia: Lippincott Williams & Wilkins, 2003.

Skeel, R.T. *Handbook of Cancer Chemotherapy,* 6th ed. Philadelphia: Lippincott Williams & Wilkins, 2003.

Index

A

Abbreviations, dangerous, 284t
ABO blood type, 202-203, 203t
Absorption, drug, 150
Access or adaptation devices, needle-free, 163
Accessory cephalic vein, 18i, 48t
Acetate in parenteral nutrition solution, 266
Acetone, urine, 263t
Acidic drugs, 152-153, 159
Active transport, 10
Adapter plug, luer-locking, 57, 65, 66i
Add-a-line sets, 38
   features of, 39, 40, 41i
   priming, 45
Additives, parenteral nutrition solution, 265, 266, 274
Administration sets, 38-39, 40-41i
   attaching, 43-44
   for central therapy, 109
   changing, 72
   infusion rates for, 22-23, 24i, 157
   piggyback, 171i
   priming, 44-46
   for transfusion, 207-208
Adults, nomogram for, 156i
Adverse effects
   of chemotherapy, 247-252
   of opioids, 179, 182

Adverse reactions
   to drugs, 153-154
   to lipid emulsions, 275
Air embolism
   in central therapy, 111, 113-114, 122-123t
   in parenteral nutrition, 279t, 280
   in peripheral therapy, 82-83t
Albumin
   osmotic force of, 11
   serum, test for, 261t
   transfusion of, 216-217t
Alcohol, cleaning site with, 84
Aldosterone, 3
Alkaline drugs, 152-153, 159
Alkaloids, plant, 232t
Alkylating drugs, 232t
Allergic or anaphylactic reactions, 154
   to chemotherapy, 245-247
   to drugs, 153, 185-187, 186t
   in peripheral therapy, 84-85t
   to transfusions, 208, 210, 221, 222-223t, 224-226
Alopecia, 247, 249, 251t
American Society of Health-System Pharmacists, 238
Amino acids in parenteral nutrition, 263, 264, 265, 266
Ammonia level, elevated, 224-225t, 227
Analgesia, patient-controlled, 178-183
Anemia, 250t

---

i refers to an illustration; t refers to a table.

Anesthetics, local, 60, 61i, 137
Antecubital veins, 18i
   stabilizing, 62t
   venipuncture in, 47, 49t, 107-108
Anthropometric measurements, 258-260
   formula for, 260t
   taking, 259i
Antibiotic antineoplastics, 232t
Antibodies
   ABO blood type, 202-203, 203t
   anti-Rh, 204
   monoclonal, 236
Antidiuretic hormone, 3
Antidotes for vesicant extravasation, 244-245, 244t
Antigens
   ABO blood type, 202-203
   anaphylaxis and, 154
   human leukocyte, 204
   Rh blood type, 204
Antihemophilic factor, 216-217t
Antihormones, 233, 233t
Antimetabolites, 232t
Arm, edematous or impaired, 46-47
Arm board, 69-70
Arm veins, 18i
   poor access to, 46-47, 153
   stabilizing, 62t
   upper, 47, 49t
Arrhythmias, 111
Arrow catheter, 99i
Arterial puncture, 125-126
Arteries, veins vs., 47, 50-51
Autologous blood, 205
Autotransfusion, 218

B

Bacteremia, 82-83t
Bacterial contamination of blood, 222-223t, 226
Bacterial phlebitis, 128

Basic (primary) sets, 38
   features of, 39, 40i
   priming, 44
Basilic vein, 18i
   central venous catheters in, 88i, 104, 105t, 107
   stabilizing, 62t
   venipuncture in, 49t
Bevacizumab, 236
Biological response modifiers, 236-238
Bladder cancer, chemotherapy for, 234t
Bleeding
   during catheter removal, 129
   at insertion site, 128
   internal, 125-126
   transfusion-related, 224-225t, 227
Blood
   composition of, 16, 196
   separating, 196
Blood-borne pathogens
   disease transmission by, 228
   protection from, 163-164, 195
Blood donors, 203, 205, 206
Blood products, 196
   guide to, 198-201t
   transfusing, 16, 196-197, 200
Blood samples
   from central venous catheter, 111, 117
   problems drawing, 119t, 120, 145t
   from vascular access port, 142
   during venipuncture, 66, 67
Blood transfusions. *See* Transfusions.
Blood type compatibility, 201-205
   ABO, 202-203, 203t
   human leukocyte antigen, 204
   Rh, 204, 205
Body fluids. *See* Fluids, body.

---

i refers to an illustration; t refers to a table.

Body surface area
  drug dosages based on, 154
  nomograms for, 155i, 156i
Body weight. *See* Weight.
Bolus doses in patient-controlled analgesia, 180-181
Bolus injection. *See* Direct injection.
Breast cancer, chemotherapy for, 234t
Broviac catheter, 90-91, 94-95t
Burette sets. *See* Volume-control sets.
Butterfly needles, 53, 55i, 57, 74

C

Calcium, 6-7t
  drug incompatibility with, 151
  in parenteral nutrition solution, 266
Calcium imbalances, 7t
  in parenteral nutrition, 278t, 282t
  in transfusions, 224-225t, 227-228
Calories
  deficiency of, 255-257
  requirements for, 253
Cancer
  chemotherapy for, 229, 234-235t. *See also* Chemotherapeutic drugs.
  immunotherapy for, 236-238
Capillary filtration and reabsorption, 10-11
Caps
  central venous catheter, changing, 117
  luer-locking, 57, 65, 66i
  vascular access port, 137
Catheter-related problems
  in central therapy, 118, 119-120t, 120
  in parenteral nutrition, 277, 278t, 279-280

Catheter-related problems
  in central therapy *(continued)*
  in peripheral therapy, 76-79t
  in vascular access port, 145t
Catheters, gauges for, 56t. *See also* Central venous catheters; Infusion devices.
Cell cycle, chemotherapeutic drugs and, 230, 231i
Cells, chemotherapy's effect on, 229
Cellular products, 196
  guide to, 198-201t
  transfusing, 16, 196-197, 200
Centers for Medicare and Medicaid Services, 29
Central venous catheters, 88-103
  changing caps on, 117
  documenting insertion of, 112
  drawing blood from, 117, 119t, 120
  dressings for, 112, 114-115i
  flushing, 115-117
  guide to, 92-97t
  insertion of, 110-111
  parenteral nutrition via, 254, 268, 271
  problems with, 118, 119-120t, 120
  removal of, 129-130
  transfusions via, 195
  vascular access ports vs., 100-101t
Central venous therapy, 86
  assisting with, 109-112
  benefits and risks of, 86-87
  catheters for, 88-103
  complications of, 87, 121-128
  documenting, 112, 117, 118, 143, 148
  equipment for, 109
  infusion problems in, 118, 119-120t, 120
  insertion sites for, 104-108
  patient monitoring for, 111

---

i refers to an illustration; t refers to a table.

Central venous therapy *(continued)*
  patient teaching for, 108
  for pediatric, elderly, and home-care patients, 120-121
  preparing for, 103-104
  routine care in, 113-117
  stopping, 128-130
  vascular access ports for, 131-148
  veins used in, 18i, 87-88, 88-89i
Cephalic vein, 18i
  central venous catheters in, 105i, 107
  stabilizing, 62t
  venipuncture in, 49t
Cervical cancer, chemotherapy for, 234t
Chemical incompatibility of drug, 151-153
Chemotherapeutic drugs, 229
  cell cycle and, 230, 231i
  complications of, 242-252
  giving, 242
  guidelines for, 238
  preparing, 238-241
  protocols for, 234-235t
  selecting, 230
  types of, 232-233t
Chemotherapy spill kit, 241
Chevron taping method, 68i
Children
  central therapy for, 88, 120-121
  drug administration for, 162, 183-184
  fluid and electrolyte imbalances in, 286-288t
  nomogram for, 155i
  parenteral nutrition for, 276-277
  transfusions for, 218-219
  vascular access ports in, 144
Chloride
  functions of, 6-7t
  in parenteral nutrition solution, 266
Chylothorax, 122-123t, 127

Circulatory overload
  in drug therapy, 186t
  in peripheral therapy, 82-83t
  in transfusions, 222-223t
Citrate toxicity, 227
Clamps, I.V., 23, 25
Class II Biological Safety Cabinet, 238-239
Clot formation
  in central therapy, 119t, 120
  in parenteral nutrition, 277, 278t
  in vascular access port, 142-143, 145t
Cold agglutinins, 208
Colloid osmotic pressure, 11
Colony-stimulating factors, 237-238
Complications
  of central therapy, 87, 111, 121-128
  of chemotherapy, 242-252
  of drug administration, 153-154, 185-193
  of parenteral nutrition, 271, 274-275, 277-282
  of patient-controlled analgesia, 182
  of peripheral therapy, 36, 74-75, 76-85t
  of transfusions, 195, 208, 210-211, 219-228
  of vascular access ports, 144, 146-147t
Concentration, drug, 152
Consent for vascular access port implantation, 135
Contact time, drug, 152
Continuous infusion, 17, 19-20, 22
  converting to intermittent, 57, 65, 66i, 129
  of drug, 166-167t, 176-178
  methods for, 19t
  of parenteral nutrition, 268, 269

---

i refers to an illustration; t refers to a table.

Continuous infusion *(continued)*
   of patient-controlled analgesia, 180-182
   phlebitis after, 191
   starting vascular access port, 139-140, 141i
Court cases, 27
Creatinine height index, 261t
Cross-sensitivity, 153
Cuffs
   on blood bag, 212i, 213
   central venous catheter, 89i, 90
CV therapy. *See* Central venous therapy.
Cycle-nonspecific chemotherapy, 230, 232t, 233
Cycle-specific chemotherapy, 230, 231i, 232-233, 232t
Cyclic total parenteral nutrition, 268, 269
Cytokines, immunomodulatory, 236-238
Cytomegalovirus, 228
Cytoprotective drugs, 233t

D

Daunorubicin, antidote for, 244t
Degranulation in anaphylaxis, 154
Delivery routes and methods, 17-22, 149-150
Dermis, 50i
Dextrose in parenteral nutrition solutions, 263, 264, 265, 266
Diagnostic studies for nutritional deficiencies, 260, 261-263t
Diarrhea, chemotherapy-related, 249
Dietary history, 258
Diffusion, 10
Digital veins, 18i, 48t
Diluents
   compatibility of, 151
   reconstituting drugs with, 158-159, 160
Diluting liquid drugs, 159-160

Dimethyl sulfoxide (DMSO), 244t
2,3-Diphosphoglycerate, 227
Direct injection, 17, 22, 164, 167
   into existing line, 169
   methods for, 21t, 165t
   phlebitis after, 191
   into vascular access port, 138-139
   into vein, 167-168
Disconnected catheter, 120t
Disease transmission
   protection from, 163-164, 195
   transfusion-related, 228
Dislodged catheter, 76-77t, 277, 278t
Documentation, 30-33
   of blood transfusion, 213
   of central catheter insertion, 112
   of central therapy, 117, 118
   of complications, 75
   of drug administration, 179
   federal regulations for, 29
   flow sheet for, 285i
   forms for, 30-32
   of infusion site complications, 243
   for I.V. bag, 33
   of I.V. insertion, 35
   of plasma transfusion, 215
   tips for, 31
   for vascular access port, 143, 148
Donors, blood, 203, 205, 206
Dosages, drug
   abbreviations for, 284t
   calculating, 154-156
   for patient-controlled analgesia, 179-182
Doxorubicin, antidote for, 244t
Dressings
   applying transparent, 67, 69i
   central venous, 112, 114-115i
   changing, 70-71
   labeling, 30, 32
Drip controllers, 109

---

i refers to an illustration; t refers to a table.

Drops per minute, calculating, 24, 157
Drugs, I.V., 16, 149. *See also* Chemotherapeutic drugs.
  abbreviations for, 284t
  adding to container, 161
  adding to primary line, 73
  adding to volume-control set, 174i, 175
  adverse reactions to, 153-154
  benefits of, 149-150
  for children, 183-184
  complications of, 185-193
  containers for, 38
  continuous infusion of, 176-178
  direct injection of, 21t, 22, 164, 167-169
  documentation for, 179
  dosages for, 154-156
  for elderly, 185
  equipment for, 161-163
  five rights for administering, 164
  immunotherapeutic, 236-238
  incompatibility of, 57, 151-153, 159
  infiltration of, 75
  infusion methods for, 164, 165-167t
  infusion rates for, 156-157
  intermittent infusion of, 169-176
  lawsuits involving, 26-28
  nurse practice acts and, 157-158
  patient-controlled administration of, 178-183
  patient preparation for, 163-164
  preparing, 158-161
  risks of, 150-154
  vascular access for, 153
Dual-lumen catheter, 57
Dual-Lumen Per-Q-Cath, 98i

E

Elderly patients
  central therapy for, 120-121
  drug administration for, 185

Elderly patients *(continued)*
  fluid and electrolyte imbalances in, 289-291t
  parenteral nutrition for, 276, 277
  peripheral therapy for, 73-74
  tourniquets on, 58-59
  transfusions for, 219
  vascular access ports in, 144
Electrolyte balance, 1, 8-9
Electrolyte imbalances, 7t, 9t
  in children, 286-287t
  in elderly, 289-290t
  in parenteral nutrition, 278-279t, 280, 281-282t
  in transfusions, 224-225t, 227-228
Electrolytes
  major, 4-5, 6-9t
  in parenteral nutrition solutions, 264, 265, 266
Electronic infusion devices, priming, 44, 45
Embolism, air. *See* Air embolism.
Enzymes, chemotherapeutic, 232t
Epidermis, 50i
Equipment
  for central therapy, 109
  for chemotherapy preparation, 238-239
  for drug administration, 161-163
  infusion rates and, 157
  for parenteral nutrition, 270, 273-274
  for peripheral therapy, 38-46
  for transfusions, 207-208, 214
  for vascular access ports, 131-133, 136
Erythrocytes, 201
Erythropoietin, 237
Extended peripheral catheter, 93, 96
External jugular vein, 18i
  catheters in, 104, 105t, 107, 108
  circulation through, 87
Extracellular fluid, 2, 2i, 8-9

---

i refers to an illustration; t refers to a table.

Extravasation
  antidotes for, 244-245, 244t
  of chemotherapeutic drug, 243-245
  of drug, 188-189, 191
  in parenteral nutrition, 271, 274, 279, 279t, 280
  preventing, 190
  of vascular access port, 146-147t

F

Facility policy, 29-30
Factors II, VII, IX, X complex, 216-217t
Factor VIII, 216-217t
Fats in parenteral nutrition solutions, 263, 264, 265. *See also* Lipid emulsions.
Febrile reactions, 221, 222-223t
Federal regulations, 28-29
Femoral veins, 18i, 106-107
Fibrin sheath formation, 120, 146-147t
Filters
  attaching, 46
  for blood transfusion, 207-208
  in-line, 39, 42
  for plasma transfusion, 214
Filtration, capillary, 10-11
Five rights of drug administration, 164
Flow sheets, 32, 285i
Fluid balance, 1-4, 8
Fluid imbalances
  in children, 288t
  correcting, 11-15
  in elderly, 290-291t
  identifying, 5
Fluids, body, 1-4
  daily gains and losses of, 4
  deficit or excess of, 5
  distribution of, 2i
  movement of, 9-11
  precautions for handling, 163-164, 193, 195

Fluid volume deficit, 5
  in children, 288t
  in elderly, 291t
Fluid volume excess, 5
  in drug therapy, 177, 186t
  in elderly, 290t
  in parenteral nutrition, 276, 277, 280
  in peripheral therapy, 82-83t
  in transfusions, 222-223t
Flushing
  central venous catheters, 115-117
  problems with, 145t
  vascular access ports, 140, 142, 144-147
Folic acid analogs, 233t
Folic acid in parenteral nutrition solutions, 266
Forearm veins, 18i, 47, 48-49t
Forms for documentation, 30-32, 285i
Fresh frozen plasma, 216-217t

G

Gastric cancer, chemotherapy for, 234t
Gauges
  needle and catheter, 56t
  noncoring needle, 134
  peripherally inserted central catheter, 91-92
Gauze dressings, changing, 70
Glass bottles, 38
  adding drug to, 161
  attaching, 43-44
  inspecting, 42-43
  tubing for, 162
Gloves and gowns for chemotherapy preparation, 239-240
Glucose balance, parenteral nutrition and, 266-267
Granulocyte colony-stimulating factor, 237

---

i refers to an illustration; t refers to a table.

Granulocyte-macrophage colony-stimulating factor, 238
Granulocytes, transfusion of, 197
Groshong catheters, 94-95t, 98i
Guide wires, peripherally inserted central catheter, 91

H

Hair loss, chemotherapy-related, 247, 249, 251t
Hand veins, 18i
  stabilizing, 62t
  venipuncture in, 47, 48t
Hazardous waste containers, chemotherapy, 239, 241
Head and neck cancer, chemotherapy for, 234t
Health care facility policy, 29-30
Hematocrit, 261t
Hematoma, 78-79t, 220
Hemiparesis of blood, 218
Hemoglobin
  increased oxygen affinity for, 224-225t, 227
  test for, 261t
Hemolytic reactions, 195, 221
  blood type incompatibility and, 201
  managing, 222-223t
  monitoring for, 208
  prevention of, 205, 207
  symptoms of, 202
Hemosiderosis, 224-225t, 226
Hemothorax, 122-123t, 125-126
Heparin flush
  for central venous catheters, 116-117
  for vascular access ports, 140, 142, 144-147
Hepatitis, 228
Hickman-Broviac catheter, 96-97t
Hickman catheter, 94-95t
Hodgkin's disease, chemotherapy for, 235t

Home-care patients
  central therapy for, 105-106, 108, 120-121
  facility policy for, 30
  parenteral nutrition for, 268, 269
  vascular access ports in, 144
Homologous blood, 205
Hormones and hormone inhibitors, 233, 233t
H taping method, 68i
Human immunodeficiency virus, 228
Human leukocyte antigens, 204
Hydrostatic pressure, 11
Hydrothorax, 122-123t, 127
Hyperalimentation, 253. *See also* Parenteral nutrition.
Hypercalcemia, 7t
Hyperchloremia, 7t
Hyperglycemia, 278t, 281t
Hyperkalemia, 7t
  in children, 286t
  in elderly, 289t
  in parenteral nutrition, 279t, 281t
  in transfusions, 224-225t, 228
Hypermagnesemia, 9t
Hypernatremia, 7t
  in children, 287t
  in elderly, 290t
Hyperosmolar hyperglycemic nonketotic syndrome, 278t
Hyperphosphatemia, 9t
Hypersensitivity reactions
  to chemotherapy, 245-247
  to drugs, 153, 185-187, 186t
  in peripheral therapy, 84-85t
  to transfusions, 208, 210, 221, 222-223t, 224-226
Hypertonic solutions, 12i, 13-14, 14-15t
Hypervolemia, 5
  in drug therapy, 177, 186t
  in elderly, 290t

---

i refers to an illustration; t refers to a table.

Hypervolemia (continued)
  in parenteral nutrition, 276, 277, 280
  in peripheral therapy, 82-83t
  in transfusions, 222-223t
Hypocalcemia, 7t
  in parenteral nutrition, 278t, 282t
  in transfusions, 224-225t, 227-228
Hypochloremia, 7t
Hypoglycemia, 266, 276, 278t, 281t
Hypokalemia, 7t
  in children, 286-287t
  in elderly, 289t
  in parenteral nutrition, 278t, 281t
Hypomagnesemia, 9t, 278t, 282t
Hyponatremia, 7t
  in children, 287t
  in elderly, 290t
Hypophosphatemia, 9t, 278t, 282t
Hypothermia, transfusion-related, 208, 224-225t, 227
Hypotonic solutions, 12i, 13, 14-15t
Hypovolemia, 5
  in children, 288t
  in elderly, 291t
Hypovolemic shock, 126

I

Iatrogenic protein-energy malnutrition, 257
Idiosyncratic drug reaction, 154
Immobilization devices, 69-70
Immune response
  in anaphylaxis, 154
  to blood type incompatibility, 202-203, 204
Immunotherapy, 236-238
Implantable pumps, 102i, 103
Implantation, vascular access port, 131, 133-136

Incompatibility
  blood type, 201-205
  drug-solution, 57, 151-153, 159
  plasma protein, 222-223t, 226
Infants. *See also* Children.
  central venous site in, 104
  drug administration for, 162, 183, 184
Infection
  in central therapy, 124-127t
  in drug therapy, 187t, 193
  parenteral nutrition-related, 271, 274, 275, 278t
  in peripheral therapy, 82-83t
  transfusion-related transmission of, 195, 228
  vascular access port site, 146-147t
Inferior vena cava, 87
Infiltration
  of chemotherapeutic drug, 242-243
  of drug, 186t, 188
  of parenteral nutrition solution, 274
  in peripheral therapy, 74-75, 76-77t
  scale for, 189t
Informed consent for vascular access port implantation, 135
Infusion devices. *See also* Central venous catheters.
  basic, 54-55i
  electronic, priming, 44, 45
  infiltration involving, 75
  inserting, 62-66
  intermittent, 57, 65, 66i
  removing, 84-85
  securing, 66-70
  selecting, 52-53, 57
  variations on, 57
Infusion line, existing
  adding drug to, 161
  direct injection into, 21t, 165t, 169

---

i refers to an illustration; t refers to a table.

Infusion Nurses Society, 30, 238
Infusion Nursing Standards of Practice, 30
Infusion pumps, 23
  in central therapy, 109
  for drug administration, 162, 175
  rate calculation for, 157
  setting up and monitoring, 46
Infusion rates, 22-26
  administration sets and, 22-23, 162
  calculating, 24i
  checking, 25-26
  drug, calculating, 156-157
  regulating, 23, 25
Infusions, central venous
  additional care for, 117-128
  routine care for, 112-117
  stopping, 128-130
Infusions, drug
  chemotherapeutic, 242
  methods for, 164-185
  preventing extravasation during, 190
Infusions, parenteral nutrition, 254, 268
  peripheral, 273-275
  stopping, 276
  total, 268-273
Infusions, peripheral
  adding to primary line, 73
  advancing catheter during, 63-64
  maintaining, 70-73
  methods for, 17-22
  preparing for, 36-57
  stopping, 84-85
  venipuncture for, 58-70
Infusions, vascular access port, 131
  documenting, 143
  giving, 136-140, 141i
  maintaining, 140, 142-143
  stopping, 144-147

Injections
  direct. *See* Direct injection.
  lidocaine, 60, 61i, 137
In-line filters, 39, 42
Insertion sites, central, 105t
  preparing, 110
  selecting, 104-108
  vascular access port, 136-138
Insertion sites, peripheral
  changing, 73
  comparing, 48-49t
  preparing, 59-62
  selecting, 46-52
Insulin, parenteral nutrition solution with, 272, 274
Insurance carriers, 29
Intake and output sheets, 32
Interferon alpha, 237
Interleukins, 237
Intermittent infusion, 17, 22
  converting continuous to, 57, 65, 66i, 129
  of drug, 162, 166t, 169-176, 183
  methods for, 20t
  of parenteral nutrition, 268, 269
  phlebitis after, 191
  via vascular access port, 131, 140
Internal jugular vein, 18i
  catheters in, 89i, 104, 105t, 106
  circulation through, 87
International unit, abbreviation for, 284t
Interstitial fluid, 2, 2i
Intracellular fluid, 2, 2i, 8-9
Intramuscular drug administration, 150, 153
Intraosseous infusion, 184
Intravascular fluid, 2, 2i
Isotonic solutions, 12i, 13, 14-15t
I.V. bags. *See* Solution containers.
I.V. drugs. *See* Chemotherapeutic drugs; Drugs, I.V.
I.V. orders. *See* Orders.

---

i refers to an illustration; t refers to a table.

I.V. push. *See* Direct injection.
I.V. solutions. *See* Solutions.
I.V. therapy, 1. *See also* Central venous therapy; Peripheral I.V. therapy.
  benefits and risks of, 3
  delivery routes and methods for, 17-22
  documentation of, 30-33
  infusion rates for, 22-26
  objectives of, 1-17
  patient teaching for, 33-34
  professional and legal standards for, 26-30

J

Joint Commission on Accreditation of Healthcare Organizations, 29-30
Jugular veins, 18i
  catheters in, 104, 105t
  circulation through, 87
  external, 107, 108
  internal, 89i, 106

K

Ketone bodies, urine, 263t
Kilocalories, 253
Kilograms, converting pounds to, 154
Kinked catheters, 118, 145t
Kwashiorkor, 257

L

Labeling
  dressings, 30, 32
  solution containers, 30, 33, 43, 160
Laboratory tests
  for blood transfusion, 201-202, 228
  for nutritional deficiencies, 260, 261-263t
Laminar airflow hood, vertical, 238-239

Legal standards, 26-30
Leukemia, chemotherapy for, 234t
Leukocyte-poor red blood cells, 197, 198-199t
Leukocytes
  transfusion of, 197, 200-201t
  in whole blood, 196
Leukopenia, 250t
Lidocaine injections, 60, 61i, 137
Ligament damage, 80-81t
Light, drug exposure to, 152, 153
Lipid emulsions, 267-268
  administering, 270
  for children, 277
  complications of, 275, 282
  concentrations for, 263, 264, 265
Liquid drugs, diluting, 159-160
Liver dysfunction, 279t
Loading dose for patient-controlled analgesia, 179, 181
Local anesthetics, 60, 61i, 137
Local complications of peripheral therapy, 74, 76-81t
Lock-out interval in patient-controlled analgesia, 179, 180, 181
Long-line catheter, 96-97t
Luer-locking cap, 57, 65, 66i
Lung cancer, chemotherapy for, 235t
Lymphocyte count, total, 262t
Lymphoma, chemotherapy for, 234t, 235t

M

Macrodrip sets, 23, 24i, 38-39
Magnesium, 8-9t
  imbalances of, 9t, 278t, 282t
  in parenteral nutrition solutions, 266
Magnesium sulfate, abbreviation for, 284t
Malignancy, secondary, 252

---

i refers to an illustration; t refers to a table.

Malnutrition, protein-energy, 256-257
Marasmus, 257
Mechanical phlebitis, 47, 128
Mechlorethamine, antidote for, 244t
Median antebrachial vein, 18i, 49t
Medicare and Medicaid, 28-29
Melanoma, chemotherapy for, 234t
Membrane, volume-control set with, 176
Metabolic acidosis, 279t
Metabolic complications of parenteral nutrition, 278t-279t, 280, 281t-282t
Metabolism, drug, 150
Metacarpal veins, 18i
   stabilizing, 62t
   venipuncture in, 47, 48t
Microaggregate filter, 207-208, 214
Microdrip sets, 23, 24i, 38-39
Micronutrients in parenteral nutrition, 264, 265, 266
Mid-arm length and mid-arm muscle circumference, 259i, 260t
Midline device, 93, 96
Milliliters-per-hour calculations, 156, 157
Minerals in parenteral nutrition, 264, 265, 266
Minibag, mixing drug in, 159
Mixing order, drug incompatibility and, 152
Monoclonal antibodies, 236
Morphine sulfate, abbreviation for, 284t
Multilumen central venous catheter, 92t-93t
Multiple myeloma, chemotherapy for, 235t
Myelosuppression, 249, 250t-251t

N

Nausea and vomiting
   chemotherapy-related, 248t-249t
   opioid-related, 182
Needleless systems, 53, 163i
Needles
   butterfly, 53, 55i, 57, 74
   for drug preparation, 158
   gauges for, 56t
   infiltration involving, 75
Needles, noncoring, 132, 133i
   choosing, 134
   inserting, 131, 132i
   problems with, 145t
   removing, 148
Nerve damage, 80t-81t
Nitrogen mustard, antidote for, 244t
Nomograms, 154, 155i, 156i
Non-Hodgkin's lymphoma, chemotherapy for, 234t
Nontunneled central venous catheters, 89-90, 92t-93t
Nonvented administration sets, 23
Nonvented bottle, attaching, 43
Nurse practice acts, 28
   drug administration and, 157-158
   transfusions and, 194
Nutrition, parenteral. *See* Parenteral nutrition.
Nutritional assessment, 257-260, 261t-263t
Nutritional deficiencies, 255-257

O

Occlusion, 78t-79t
Occupational Safety and Health Administration, 238
Oncology Nursing Society, 238
Oncotic pressure, 11
Opioid analgesics, 178-183
Oral drugs, absorption of, 150

---

i refers to an illustration; t refers to a table.

Orders
  additional, calculations for, 157
  for parenteral nutrition, 270-271, 274
  reading, 27
OSHA. *See* Occupational Safety and Health Administration.
Osmolarity
  in I.V. solutions, 11, 12i, 13-15
  serum, 11
Osmosis, 10, 11
Output, documentation of, 32
Over-the-needle catheters, 53, 54i
  advancing, 64
  inserting, 63
  vascular access port, 133

P

Packed red blood cells, 197, 198-199t
Pain
  I.V. drug-related, 150
  at I.V. site, 78-79t, 128
Parenteral nutrition, 16-17, 253
  for children and elderly, 276-277
  complications of, 277-282
  elements in, 16, 253
  giving, 268-275
  indications for, 254-255
  infusion methods for, 254
  lipid emulsions in, 270
  nutritional assessment for, 257-260, 261-263t
  reducing infection risk in, 271
  solutions for, 263-268
  stopping, 276
  switching from continuous to cyclic, 269
  via vascular access port, 131
Partial parenteral nutrition. *See* Peripheral parenteral nutrition.
Pathogens, blood-borne
  disease transmission by, 228
  protection from, 163-164, 195

Patient-controlled analgesia, 178-183
  complications of, 182
  evaluating pump for, 180
  managing, 180-182
  patient teaching for, 182-183
Patient monitoring
  after central venous catheter insertion, 111
  after vascular access port implantation, 136
Patient positioning for central venous catheter insertion, 108, 110
Patient preparation
  for drug administration, 163-164
  for parenteral nutrition, 269, 273
  for peripheral therapy, 36-38
  for vascular access port implantation, 134-135
Patient teaching, 33-34
  for patient-controlled analgesia, 182-183
  for peripheral therapy, 37
  reinforcing central therapy, 108
PCA. *See* Patient-controlled analgesia.
Pediatric patients. *See* Children.
Penicillin, anaphylactic reactions to, 153, 154
Peripheral I.V. therapy, 35-36
  adding infusions in, 73
  basics of, 36
  complications of, 74-75, 76-85t, 186-187t
  documentation for, 35, 75
  for elderly patients, 73-74
  equipment selection and preparation for, 38-46
  infusion devices for, 52-57
  insertion site for, 46-52
  patient preparation for, 36-38
  routine care in, 70-73
  stopping, 84-85

---

i refers to an illustration; t refers to a table.

Peripheral I.V. therapy *(continued)*
   veins used in, 18i, 47, 48-49t, 50-52
   venipuncture for, 58-70
Peripherally inserted central catheters, 91-93, 96
   advantages and disadvantages of, 96-97, 100
   complications of, 128
   guide to, 98-99i
Peripheral parenteral nutrition, 17. *See also* Parenteral nutrition.
   for children and elderly, 277
   complications of, 282
   giving, 273-275
   indications for, 255
   infusion method for, 254
   solutions for, 265t, 267-268
   stopping, 276
Peripheral veins, 18i
   central venous catheters in, 87-88, 88i, 107-108
   parenteral nutrition via, 254
   transfusions via, 195
Per-Q-Cath, 98i
pH, drug incompatibility and, 152-153, 159
Phlebitis
   bacterial, 128
   detecting and classifying, 192
   in drug therapy, 187t, 191-193
   mechanical, 47, 128
   in parenteral nutrition, 279t, 280
   in peripheral therapy, 76-77t
Phosphate in parenteral nutrition solutions, 266
Phosphorus
   functions of, 8t
   imbalances of, 9t, 278t, 282t
Physical assessment of nutritional status, 258
Physical incompatibility of drug, 151
PICC. *See* Peripherally inserted central catheters.

Piggyback method, 20t, 166t
   for drug administration, 170-171
   in peripheral therapy, 73
   setting up set for, 171i
   Y-site for, 22
Plant alkaloids, 232t
Plasma, 2i, 196
Plasma products
   documentation for, 215
   guide to, 216-217t
   transfusion of, 213-215
Plasma protein incompatibility, 222-223t, 226
Plasma substitutes, 214
Plastic bags, 38
   adding drug to, 161
   attaching, 44
   inspecting, 42-43
   tubing for, 162
Plastic catheter sets, 53, 54i, 75
Platelets
   transfusion of, 200-201t
   in whole blood, 196
Pneumothorax
   in central therapy, 121, 122-123t, 124-125, 128
   in parenteral nutrition, 278t, 280
Postoperative care of vascular access port, 135
Potassium
   functions of, 6t
   in parenteral nutrition solutions, 266
Potassium imbalances, 7t
   in children, 286-287t
   in elderly, 289t
   in parenteral nutrition, 278t, 279t, 281t
   in transfusions, 224-225t, 228
Pounds-to-kilograms conversion, 154
Powdered drugs, reconstituting, 158-159, 160
PPN. *See* Peripheral parenteral nutrition.

---

i refers to an illustration; t refers to a table.

Prealbumin, 263t
Pregnancy, managing Rh, 205
Preservatives, drug, 153
Pressure cuff on blood bag, 212i, 213
Primary line
  adding piggyback to, 73, 170-171, 171i
  basic sets for, 38, 39, 40i
  continuous infusion via, 19t
  drug infusion via, 166-167t, 176-177
  priming, 44
  volume-control set used as, 173-176
Priming administration sets, 44-46
Professional standards, 26-30
Prostate cancer, chemotherapy for, 234t
Protective clothing for chemotherapy preparation, 239-240
Protein-calorie deficiency, 255-256
Protein-energy malnutrition, 256-257
Protein screen, total, 262t
Prothrombin complex, 216-217t
Protocols, chemotherapy, 234-235t
Pumps. *See also* Infusion pumps.
  implantable, 102i, 103
  patient-controlled analgesia, 178-182
  syringe, 184

Q
Q.d. versus q.o.d., 284t

R
Rate minder, 25
Reabsorption, capillary, 10-11
Reconstituting powdered drugs, 158-159, 160
Red blood cells
  transfusion of, 197, 198-199t
  in whole blood, 196
Reimbursement, 28-29
Reservoirs, vascular access port, 131-132
Respiratory depression, 179, 182
Retrograde administration, 184
Rh blood type, 204, 205
Right-angle noncoring needle, 133i, 134
Rights of drug administration, 164
Rituximab, 236
Roller clamp, 23
Routes of administration, 17, 18i, 149-150
Routine care
  in central therapy, 113-117
  in peripheral therapy, 70-73

S
Safety precautions
  for chemotherapy preparation, 240-241
  for drug preparation, 158, 159
  for total parenteral nutrition, 272
Saline flush
  for central venous catheters, 115-117
  for vascular access ports, 140, 142, 144-147
Saline lock, 20t, 166t
  converting to, 57, 66i
  equipment for, 172-173
  hints for handling, 173
  using, 65, 172i
Screening tests for blood, 201-202, 228
Screw clamp, 23
Secondary line
  administration sets for, 38, 39, 40, 41i
  central venous infusion via, 117
  continuous infusion via, 19t

---

i refers to an illustration; t refers to a table.

Secondary line *(continued)*
  drug infusion via, 167t, 170-171, 177-178
  priming, 45
  volume-control set used as, 174-176
Secondary malignancy, 252
Sepsis
  in central therapy, 126-127t, 127-128
  in parenteral nutrition, 274, 275, 278t
  in peripheral therapy, 82-83t
Sequential numbering system, 31
Serum albumin, 261t
Serum transferrin, 262t
Serum triglycerides, 262t
Severed catheter, 78-79t
Side-entry vascular access port, 131, 137
Single-lumen central venous catheter, 92-93t
Skin, anatomy of, 50i
Skin breakdown, 146-147t
Skin-fold thickness, triceps, 259i, 260t
Slide clamp, 23
Sodium, 6-7t
  imbalances of, 7t, 287t, 290t
  in parenteral nutrition solutions, 266
Sodium thiosulfate, 244t
Solution containers, 38
  adding drug to, 161
  attaching, 43-44
  inspecting, 42-43
  labeling, 30, 33, 43, 160
  tubing for, 162
Solutions, 14-15t
  changing central, 113-115
  changing peripheral, 71-72
  delivery routes and methods for, 17-22
  drug, preparing, 158-160

Solutions *(continued)*
  drug incompatibility with, 57, 151-153, 159
  flushing, 115-117
  infusion problems with, 118, 119t
  infusion rates for, 22-26
  inspecting and preparing, 42-43
  lawsuits involving, 26-28
  osmolarity of, 11, 12i, 13
  parenteral nutrition, 16, 253, 263-268
Speed shock, 164, 167, 187t
State nurse practice acts, 28
  drug administration and, 157-158
  transfusions and, 194
Steel needles
  infiltration involving, 75
  winged, 53, 55i, 57, 74
Steroids, chemotherapeutic, 233, 233t
Stomatitis, 251-252
Straight noncoring needle, 133i, 134
Stretching technique for stabilizing veins, 62t
Stretch net, 69
Subclavian vein
  catheters in, 88-89i, 105t, 106
  circulation through, 87
Subcutaneous drug administration, 150, 153
Subcutaneous tissue, 50i
Superior vena cava
  catheters in, 87-88, 88-89i
  location of, 18i
Symbols, dangerous, 284t
Syringe pump, 184
Syringes
  drug preparation in, 158
  for peripherally inserted central catheter, 92

i refers to an illustration; t refers to a table.

Systemic complications
  of central therapy, 121, 126-127t, 127-128
  of peripheral therapy, 74, 82-85t

T

Taping techniques, 67, 68i
Teaching, patient. *See* Patient teaching.
Temperature, drug incompatibility and, 152
Tendon damage, 80-81t
Tension pneumothorax, 124-125
Testicular cancer, chemotherapy for, 235t
Therapeutic incompatibility of drug, 153
Thrombocytes, 196
Thrombocytopenia, 251t
Thrombolytics, 142, 143
Thrombophlebitis, 80-81t
Thrombosis
  in central therapy, 124-125t
  in parenteral nutrition, 279t, 280
  in peripheral therapy, 80-81t
  in vascular access port, 146-147t
Thyroid-stimulating hormone, parenteral nutrition solution with, 274
Time tape, using, 25
Titration, drug, 150
Top-entry vascular access port, 131, 132i, 137, 138i
Total lymphocyte count, 262t
Total nutrient admixture, 265-266, 267
Total parenteral nutrition, 16-17. *See also* Parenteral nutrition.
  for children and elderly, 276-277
  complications of, 277-280, 281-282t
  giving, 268-273
  handling hazards of, 278-279t
  indications for, 254-255

Total parenteral nutrition (*continued*)
  infusion method for, 254
  lipid emulsions in, 270
  precautions when maintaining, 272
  reducing infection risk in, 271
  solutions for, 264t, 265-267
  stopping, 276
  switching from continuous to cyclic, 269
  via vascular access port, 131
Total protein screen, 262t
Tourniquets, applying, 58-59, 74
Trace elements in parenteral nutrition, 264, 265, 266
Transdermal analgesic cream, 60, 137
Transferrin, serum, 262t
Transfusion reactions, 219-228
  managing, 219-221, 222-225t
  monitoring for, 208, 210-211
  multiple, 226-228
  signs or symptoms of, 211
  types of, 221, 224-226
Transfusions, 194
  blood donors for, 205, 206
  blood products for, 196, 198-201t
  blood type compatibility for, 201-205
  of cellular products, 196-197, 200
  for children and elderly, 218-219
  complex, 218
  complications of, 219-228
  correcting problems during, 220
  disease transmission in, 195, 228
  documenting, 213, 215
  "don'ts" for, 211
  equipment for, 207-208
  methods for, 195
  monitoring, 208, 210-213
  plasma and plasma fraction, 213-215, 216-217t

---

i refers to an illustration; t refers to a table.

Transfusions (*continued*)
  preparation for, 205, 207
  pressure cuff for, 212i, 213
  purposes of, 16, 194-195
  risks of, 195
  starting, 208, 209-210i
  stopping, 213
Transparent dressings
  applying, 67, 69i
  changing, 70-71
Transthyretin, 263t
Trastuzumab, 236
Traumatic complications of central therapy, 121, 122-125t, 124-127
Trendelenburg position, 108, 110
Triceps skin-fold thickness, 259i, 260t
Triglycerides, serum, 262t
Tubing
  central venous, changing, 113-115, 116
  cracked or broken, 278t
  for drug administration, 162
  kinked vascular access port, 145t
Tumor necrosis factor, 237
Tunicae intima, media, and adventitia, 51i
Tunneled central venous catheters, 90-91, 94-97t
Typing and crossmatching blood, 201-202

U

Unit, abbreviation for, 284t
Universal donor or recipient, 203
Urine ketone bodies, 263t
U taping method, 68i

V

Valsalva maneuver, 111, 113-114, 129
Valves in veins, 52
Vascular access, poor, 153

Vascular access ports, 100-101
  advantages and disadvantages of, 103
  blood samples from, 142
  central venous catheters versus, 100-101t
  clearing, 142-143
  common problems with, 145t
  complications of, 144, 146-147t
  documentation for, 143, 148
  equipment for, 131-133, 136
  flushing, 140, 142, 144-147
  giving infusions via, 131, 136-140, 141i
  implantation of, 131, 133-136
  interrupting therapy via, 144-148
  maintaining infusions via, 140, 142-143
  preventing problems with, 143-144
Vein flare, 245
Veins
  anatomy of, 51i
  arteries versus, 47, 50-51
  for central therapy, 87-88, 88-89i, 104-108
  commonly used, 17, 18i, 47, 48-49t
  deep, inserting device into, 65-66
  dilating, 58-59
  direct injection into, 21t, 165t, 167-168
  inaccessible, 153
  irritation of, 78-79t
  selection guidelines for, 46-47, 52
  stabilizing, 60-61, 62t
Venipuncture
  blood samples during, 66, 67
  dilating vein for, 58-59
  for elderly patients, 73-74
  equipment for, 38-46

---

i refers to an illustration; t refers to a table.

Venipuncture (*continued*)
  inserting infusion device in, 62-66
  local anesthetic for, 60, 61i
  patient preparation for, 36-38
  poor access for, 153
  securing infusion device in, 66-70
  site preparation for, 59-62
  site selection for, 46-52
  stabilizing veins for, 62t
  Venipuncture devices. *See* Infusion devices.
Venipuncture sites. *See* Insertion sites, central; Insertion sites, peripheral.
Venogram, 135
Venous spasm, 80-81t, 187t
Vented administration sets, 22-23
Vented bottle, attaching, 43-44
Vesicant drugs, extravasation of, 188-191, 243-245
Vitamins in parenteral nutrition, 264, 265, 266
Volume-control sets, 20t, 38, 166t
  adding drugs to, 174i, 175
  for children, 162, 183
  drug infusion via, 173-176
  features of, 39, 40, 41i
  labeling, 30, 43
Vomiting
  chemotherapy-related, 248-249t
  opioid-related, 182

WX

Water
  body, 3-4
  in parenteral nutrition solution, 264
Weight
  body surface area and, 155i, 156i
  drug dosages based on, 154
  fluid balance and, 3
  fluid component of, 1, 2i

White blood cells
  transfusion of, 197, 200-201t
  in whole blood, 196
Whole blood
  components of, 16, 196
  transfusion of, 197, 198-199t
Winged infusion sets, 53, 57
  advancing, 64
  for elderly, 74
  inserting, 63
  with steel needle, 55i
  variations on, 57
Workspace for chemotherapy preparation, 238-239
Wrist veins, 18i
  catheters over, 47
  stabilizing, 62t

YZ

Y-shaped winged infusion set, 57
Y-sites
  infusion via, 22
  sets with, 39, 40i, 41i, 171i

---

i refers to an illustration; t refers to a table.